PRAISE FOR LYNN WEIMAR AND
BE FREE BEYOND FIFTY

"Lynn is a powerful and positive force! She has boldly upgraded her own life and can help anyone else do the same. This book will set you free and give you strength and courage you didn't know you had."

— **Dr. Benjamin Hardy, Organizational Psychologist and Author of *Willpower Doesn't Work* and *Personality Isn't Permanent***

"Lynn is excellent at helping those around her to become empowered now and hopeful toward their desired future. She can help you navigate the path ahead toward living life to the fullest."

— **Natasha Schiffman, Accountability Coach**

"Lynn Weimar's *Be Free Beyond Fifty* was the perfect book for me since I just turned fifty. It helped me reshape my thoughts to see that I have a lot of life left to live and I can make healthy choices so that my future can be as enjoyable as possible. After reading this book, I'm learning to reduce the size of my meals to better suit my aging body so it can perform optimally and keep me free and happy for many years to come."

— **Tyler R. Tichelaar, PhD and Award-Winning Author of *Narrow Lives* and *The Best Place***

"Lynn Weimar is an inspiration. Her Wellness Wednesdays have given me a lot of insight and encouragement into my journey and how to continue on it when life doesn't always work out. She is caring and down to earth. I am so grateful I found her and recommend her to anyone who is on this journey called life."

—**Kathy G., Sarasota, Florida**

"Before I found Lynn's program, I was at my wit's end. I was not feeling well and was having difficulty breathing. I was experiencing anxiety and lack of stamina and energy. I just didn't feel healthy. But in Lynn's program I started to experience new energy, less fatigue, more stamina. Rather than having food delivered to my home, I've been able to prepare healthy meals on my own with Lynn's help and the help of the group. That black cloud hanging over me is now gone. I have so much more confidence than I ever thought I could have. There's no more 'I'll try' or 'I hope.' It's changed to *'I will,'* because I know I can. I've got the tools."

— **Martha K., Manchester, Connecticut**

"I had gone through a very bad divorce and was having extreme financial difficulties. I needed support. When I first saw Lynn's ad, emotional eating was the least of my problems, but I felt it was a deeper program than the average and Lynn had knowledge to share beyond the norm. When I began Lynn's program, I received the help I needed, and I was able to tap into inner strength and get past any fear that had been holding me back. Now I like that I'm just facing the normal stresses of day-to-day life. I don't look at food as an adversary. I look at food as a friend. Food doesn't control me; I control food. I'm now kinder to myself and more self-forgiving."

— **Carole W., Marvell, Arkansas**

"I'm grateful to Lynn for her encouraging words on our calls and wonderful wisdom on her Facebook messages! We all struggle in life from time to time, and her support and encouragement have meant so much to me."

—**Sharon S., St. Louis, Missouri**

"Lynn's program was different than all the others I had tried because there was a lot more focus on my emotional thinking. I realized how events and my beliefs about the past affected my food choices and led to food or sugar addiction. Being able to focus more on that made a lot of difference. An unexpected shift that took place was noticing how my negative thought process was affecting not only how I felt emotionally but also the foods I chose to eat. If I was really into more negative thinking, then I would tend not to eat healthy foods. When I focus on positives, and being grateful, overall my food choices tend to be healthier. My life now is a whole lot better than I had previously thought possible."

— **Janice S., Shelbyville, Illinois**

"My life used to be so out of control. I was looking for something different than I had tried before. Lynn helped me see things from a different perspective. What I learned was that I was worth it. I now have hope, and I am so much happier. My relationship with food is so different now. I am planning and preparing ahead of time and trying new healthy food. I've ended my relationship with Mr. McDonald and Miss Wendy. Now, instead of stopping for fast food, I just speed on by. I'm breaking it off. I know I'm going to succeed. I've lost sixty pounds. And it's staying off. I will be doing this forever and ever."

— **Regina C., Welch, West Virginia**

"Before beginning coaching with Lynn, I was really unhealthy and lethargic. I looked for different solutions and tried different things. Nothing seemed to work, year after year. Every time I lost weight, it just came back on and then some. After a short time working with Lynn, I began to notice just how far I could walk without wheezing. Another big change was being able to give up the sugar in favor of fresh fruit, knowing I would be just fine with fruit. I hadn't realized the extent to which sugar addiction played a role. I also found I could look at things more logically and let go of ideas that were keeping me stuck. I immediately started feeling better. I found my voice and let go of anxiety."

— Terri L., Federal Way, Washington

"At nearly sixty years old, I had settled into the belief I never could really make any lasting changes for the better. I had been trying to gain control of my eating habits, spending habits, lazy habits as well as the fears continually keeping me from experiencing new, potentially wonderful adventures. Lynn's personal experience and wisdom stirred up new hope in me. It took me a while to completely commit to Lynn's coaching and put my trust in her direction, but I am so thankful I made that uncomfortable leap of faith. My life has changed tremendously. I no longer hope for something better; I accept something better as my reality. It is happening and I am loving the total transformation taking place within me. I am more excited about my future than I've ever been before."

— Virginia A., Boise, Idaho

"Lynn can help you discover the deep-rooted reasons for your emotional eating patterns and why you are not achieving the level of wellbeing you want. Now, I understand I eat out of boredom or worry about whatever stressful situation is going on at the time. With Lynn's assistance, I am learning how to take small steps of action with loads of compassion for myself. I encourage you to call Lynn today. It can change your life and help you find true compassion for yourself, your health, and wellbeing. I'm so grateful for Lynn giving me the encouragement to pursue my hopes and dreams for my health and life! Thank you, Lynn!"

— Melissa E., Kennesaw, Georgia

"When I started on my weight-loss journey, I knew I needed to find some place where I could share my journey, triumphs, and struggles with other women like me who were committed to being fit and being fifty. That's when I found Lynn Weimar and the Be Fit Beyond Fifty group. I finally had a place where I could share about my journey and know there were other women like me who had the same struggles. Lynn was very supportive and welcoming, and in my initial connection with her we talked about goals and dreams and possible paths to get there. This set me on my way to fulfilling my ultimate dream of taking my weight off and continuing to be able to love myself and love the person I was becoming. It's an amazing and diverse group of women who all share the same amazing goal of living to be fit and healthy. Thank you so much, Lynn, for this amazing group."

—**Mara P., Derry, New Hampshire**

"I discovered Be Fit Beyond Fifty on Facebook and was interested in what it was about, so I joined and watched the 'live' with Lynn Weimar and was instantly interested in her talks. Wow! I thought. I finally found a motivational speaker and a group of ladies my age who understand me. Yes! I *do* have a promising future! I *do* have hope for a healthy and contented life, regardless of the stresses I encounter every day. I *did* put my time in, and now it's time for *me*! So, thank you, Lynn, for being my inspiration, my motivator, and my friend on my new future journey! I am thankful I found you. You have made me realize I am worth it!"

— **Lori P., Laurel, Mississippi**

be FREE beyond fifty

Stop Hiding
Unlock Your Dream
and Step into a Vibrant Life

LYNN WEIMAR

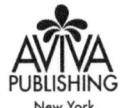

AVIVA
PUBLISHING
New York

Be Free Beyond Fifty:
Stop Hiding, Unlock Your Dream, and Step into a Vibrant Life
Copyright © 2021 by Lynn Weimar

Published by:
Aviva Publishing
Lake Placid, NY
(518) 523-1320
www.AvivaPubs.com

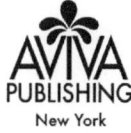

All rights reserved, including the right to reproduce this book or any portion thereof in any form whatsoever. For information, address:

Lynn Weimar
lynn@befitbeyondfifty.com
BeFitBeyondFifty.com

Every attempt has been made to source all quotes properly.

Names of individuals have been changed to protect their privacy.

For additional copies or bulk purchases, visit:
www.BeFreeBeyondFifty.com

Editor: Tyler Tichelaar, Superior Book Productions
Publishing Coach: Christine Gail
Cover Design and Interior Layout: Fusion Creative Works
Author Photo: Anna Gorin

Library of Congress Control Number: 2021911812
Hardcover ISBN: 978-1-63618-117-2
E-book ISBN: 978-1-63618-118-9

10 9 8 7 6 5 4 3 2 1
First Edition, 2021
Printed in the United States of America

To Terri, my beautiful sister.

I am thrilled beyond words watching you step into your vibrant life.

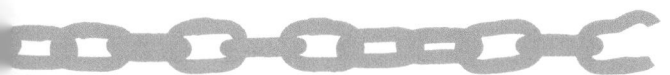

Contents

Introduction	13
Chapter 1: A Woman of Tremendous Worth	19
Chapter 2: Are You Hiding?	29
Chapter 3: Daring to Hope Again	51
Chapter 4: Accepting Where We Are Right Now	65
Chapter 5: Learning to Be Present	77
Chapter 6: Turning Our Stories Upside Down	95
Chapter 7: Valuing Ourselves Means Living in Joy	115
Chapter 8: Taking It with You	131
A Final Note: Opportunity over Impossibility	143
Acknowledgments	147
About the Author	149
Be Set Free to Live Your Best Life	151

Introduction

"You are enough." Wait. What? I allowed the words to flow over me as the tears began to flow down my face. My mind didn't quite grasp them, but my heart drank them in thirstily. I was sitting in a therapist's office. He continued, "You are smart enough, kind enough, thoughtful enough, pretty enough. You are enough. I'm not your father, but if you were my daughter, this is what I would want you to know. This is what I believe about you."

I didn't argue. I didn't try to explain away or dismiss the words by telling myself that of course he would say that, because I was paying him. No, I heard the sincerity in his voice, and I could tell he understood something about me I needed to hear but was unable to grasp on my own.

I had made this appointment at the recommendation of a friend who saw the very stuck place I was in. The therapist required background information prior to the appointment. As I set out to write this book's introduction, I thought I might still have the introductory email I wrote to him more than a decade ago buried in my sent folder. Sure enough, it was there. As I read it over again, I could hear the pain of that hurt and frightened woman. I'm filled with wonder and gratitude at just how far she has come.

Here is an excerpt from that email:

> I have spent a lot of time in the past nine months grieving the loss of my home and family. My kids understand because they have all lived through it, and they are all very supportive of me. But still, I can't help but feel like I have failed. Nobody who knows me or the circumstances is telling me to go back to my husband and try again. They are all telling me this is not my fault and I am not a failure. I've got lots of great support in my friends and family, and I am seeing another Christian counselor [name omitted], who has been helpful to me. But I feel very stuck in this area in particular, and immobilized in the rest of my life, also. Many people have told me I exhibit characteristics of an emotionally abused woman just in my demeanor. I would like to rise above that and learn what it's like to feel "normal."
>
> A little bit more about me: bachelor's degree in English, built a couple of home businesses related to home education and then transcription, editing, desktop publishing, teaching, and tutoring. Started working out and running about thirteen years ago after sixteen years of pretty much either being pregnant or nursing babies. Loved running so much that I started racing and have done about 35-40 races, mostly triathlons and long distance running (Robie nine times, five marathons, etc.). Got my personal trainer certification and spent a few years being a running coach for a women's fitness apparel store. I recently made the decision to go into nursing, and I am taking prereq classes at CWI. I hope to apply to CWI's nursing program this spring.

I am currently working full time as a CNA at [name omitted], gaining experience for my nursing career. I think what I'm best at is taking care of people. I'm hoping to use my nursing degree in helping to set up medical clinics in Third World countries and serving in short-term missions, while having a career that will pay well enough to support me in that.

People tell me I'm good at everything I try. But I would like to stop feeling like a failure, and I would like to not feel so "stuck" all the time. I'm looking forward to meeting with you tomorrow.

As he spoke with me, Dr. H, as he liked to be called, pulled up that email on his computer and read aloud to me the paragraph starting with "a little bit more about me." "Lynn," he said, "these are not the words of someone who is stuck."

Okay, I get it. I didn't sound stuck, but I knew I was. I couldn't seem to get myself out of it, no matter how hard I tried. But that day in Dr. H's office was a turning point for me. I started embracing my "enoughness." I listened on repeat to the CD he recorded for me that day in his office. I let his message to me sink deeply into my bones. I began to heal.

I have come so far since that day. I did get accepted into nursing school, and I graduated at the age of fifty-three. I remarried and started a new life and a new career. I even got my master of science degree in nursing at the age of fifty-seven.

I still hope to pursue my dream of medical missions at some point. But only a week or so after we were married eight years ago, my new husband, Ross, fell ill with end-stage renal disease. He is a paraplegic, and the combined effects of the paralysis and dialysis treatments led to multiple lengthy hospital stays and near-death incidents. Now, besides being his wife, I am also his caregiver, performing hemodialysis treatments at home four days a week.

Many of my friends and family members consider me tied down, but I know I'm free. I'm free on the inside, the only place it really matters. I understand my worth. I am in love with my life. I don't dread my days. I live each one in a state of abundance and gratitude.

And now it's my mission in life, no matter what else I want to accomplish, to help other women over fifty to experience freedom for themselves. I'm finding that it's a pretty rare thing to be free.

If you're feeling stuck, as I was for many years, and you can't see your way out, you've come to the right place. I invite you to come along with me on a journey to discover what it means to be free.

This book is intended to be interactive. I have included questions throughout to help you engage with the message and allow it to become a part of you. You don't have to have gone through anything similar to what I have experienced to find benefit in this book. Each of us has a path that's all our own. Every woman's story is unique. The one common denominator for all the women I talk to is the feeling of being stuck. If we are stuck, it means we're not free to live our best lives. That's how I felt. It didn't matter that I didn't look like I was stuck. I knew, on the inside (and I didn't have to go very deep inside to find it), that "stuck" didn't begin to describe it.

For most women I talk to, being stuck takes the form of extra pounds. This is not a book about weight loss because the extra weight we carry more often than not is merely a symptom of something deeper that's going on. Dieting, in whatever form, just addresses the symptom. It's like taking Tylenol for a fever. A fever is part of the body's immune response. It's a signal that something's going on under the surface. In just the same way, when we go out searching for the latest and greatest diet plan but still have all the internal baggage we've carried around for years, we are only treating the symptom that's appearing on the surface. If we do that, we are destined to add that latest plan to the long list of dieting disasters.

You weren't meant to be sentenced to a life in prison, no matter what your prison happens to be. You weren't meant to be stuck.

As you embark on this journey, my hope is you will start to explore what is keeping you stuck just as I did that day in Dr. H's office. I hope you will grab hold of what you learn here and do what it takes to live a life of freedom, joy, peace, and gratitude. I hope you will begin to understand you are worth it. I hope you will step fully into your very best life and begin to shine as the beautiful woman you were meant to be.

Let's begin this journey to becoming free beyond fifty!

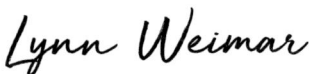

Chapter 1

A Woman of Tremendous Worth

I didn't always believe I was a woman of tremendous worth. That understanding has been gradually growing on me. And it has nothing to do with me suddenly getting a makeover, or winning a million dollars, or having plastic surgery.

I have experienced a growing realization that my worth comes from the inside. I knew this intellectually, but it never really sunk in at a deep level until I reached my mid-fifties. I could see the wrinkles and the gray hairs increasing, the weight around my middle creeping on, and the diets that were supposed to take it off just not cutting it. I still wrestled with the devastation of a failed marriage and broken family.

You may be in some of those places, too, or other places all your own. You may be wondering if life has anything left to offer you, now that you're past age fifty. Our society places a high value on outward, physical beauty, especially in women. The young, thin, and beautiful are glamorized and placed up on a pedestal. They are the sought-after ones whose pictures end up on the magazine covers. All the attention is on them, and all the opportunities come their way. At least, that's what it looks like from the outside.

And then there are the rest of us. Maybe you were one of the beautiful people back in your youth, but now that you're creeping up to fifty or even past it, you're scrambling to keep up that image. Maybe, like me, you never felt you were there in the first place. I remember thinking, as I was approaching my mid-fifties, "I wasn't pretty when I was young, so what hope is there for me now?" My only consolation was that everyone else around me, everyone else in the world, for that matter, was also aging at the same rate.

At that time, I felt more than a little beaten down by life. I still played in my head the words that had been spoken over me so many times—that I didn't measure up as a human being, that something was inherently wrong with me. Nobody had said anything like that to me in several years, but all the words kept replaying in my mind, and no matter how hard I tried, I couldn't get them out of my head.

I want to make it clear right from the beginning that I don't blame anyone for the state I was in. You know the old question, "If a tree falls in the forest and there's nobody there to hear it, does it make a noise?" Well, in the same way, radio waves are all around us, but if we don't have the receiver to pick them up, they are silent. Whatever way I was treated in the past, whether in my childhood, in college, in my marriage, or in any other relationships, only stuck to me because my receiver was turned on.

I don't blame myself for that, but I can't blame anyone else, either. I'm not going to go into any kind of diatribe about "bad things that have happened to me." I never dreamed I would end up divorced, but it happened. All the replaying I did in my head was my attempt to make sense out of it all, and to validate to myself that that's what needed to happen. Now, I'm immensely grateful for *everything* that's happened to me. I can't harbor any ill feelings toward anyone, only gratitude. I don't *want* to live there, in that stuck place of replaying past wrongs.

But that's where I was. I thought I was devalued. I thought I was silenced. I thought my voice didn't matter. Now I know that nobody did that to me; I did it to myself. I don't beat myself up for that; it's just what happened. Everything I will tell you is for the purpose of your healing. I want you to come into the place of wholeness I've been finding for myself. I'm still on the path, and I want more. I want more for you, too.

I'm in a very different place now than I've ever been in at any other time. I've come into a place of wholeness and healing. I am joyful and grateful. I don't resent anyone. I'm free. I'm at peace inside of myself and with others. That doesn't mean I've arrived or I think I'm perfect. Actually, I have so much less of a need to cling to perfectionism than I did before. I care much less about messing up. I'm free to be the best version of me. And I'm even free to be the not-so-great version of me because I've learned how to pick myself back up, forgive myself, and move on. Without shame. Without self-condemnation.

The thing I love most about all this, besides just the ability to purely enjoy my life, is I get to share what I've learned with other women (and sometimes men, too) and watch them experience the same freedom I've found.

In my work as a mindset coach and the founder of Be Fit Beyond Fifty, I have set out on a path of helping women set themselves free from emotional eating, food addictions, and a lifetime of accumulated habit patterns around food. I've talked in depth with dozens, if not hundreds, of women about these issues. I'd say a majority of them have one thing in common: they feel as if they're alone. They're locked in a prison of shame and secrecy. Many of them are shocked to hear that I talk to women nearly every day, each of whom also thinks she's the only one with the deep, dark secret of addiction and the self-loathing that goes along with it.

Many of these women have all but given up hope. They don't see anything ahead besides more failure, just like they have already experienced thousands of times before. Imagine being sentenced to life in prison. There's no parole, and no way out. Except that in this case, it's a food prison, a body prison, or a prison of shame. If that's you, I want you to know there's a way to be free. No matter how stuck you feel you are, or how many times you've tried and failed to get out of this prison on your own, there is hope for you. Yes, you.

You really can be free. You can be free to live your life the way you want to live it, without being constantly pulled on by cravings or addictions, shame or guilt, or regret. There's a way out of the prison you're in.

What does it mean to be free? Sometimes when we're caught in a web of addiction, we can't imagine life without that thing we're addicted to. The thought of never again eating a cookie or having a glass of wine, or of having to break up with social media, can send us into a tailspin.

But when I think about being free, I think about nothing pulling on me. Nothing having control over me. Being free to make my own decisions and think for myself, without having my decisions made for me by that thing that was controlling me. When I'm free, it means I don't have to live in shame or regret. I'm not beating myself up anymore, because I am in control of my own destiny. It means I'm free to embrace me, exactly as I am, right in this moment. And I'm free to reach for an even brighter future for myself. I'm not just surviving anymore. When I look in the mirror, I'm free to love what I see. I can love my body as it is and be grateful for the marvel it is.

I get to nourish my body with healthy, nutritious food and not feel like I'm missing out. I'm not needing to turn to food to numb out or feed the sugar monster that's always demanding more. I'm free to live my life exactly the way I want it to be. I can live life on my terms and love every minute of it.

A LOOK IN THE MIRROR

Are you ready for that kind of a life? I know it might sound foreign right now. And it starts with something that may sound pretty scary: taking a good, hard look in the mirror.

I don't mean the mirror you've been looking into all your life, seeing the outward, physical manifestation of you and feeling like you're coming up short. This is a mirror for taking a look at what's happening on the inside. This is the shame and blame mirror. The coping mirror. The "just help me survive this day" mirror. The "beat myself up" mirror. I'm not telling you to look in this mirror in order to do any of these things. You've had quite enough of all that, I think.

No, this is a mirror of reckoning. This is the mirror to help you begin to understand, for you and you alone, what you have been clutching as a security blanket to help you get through another day.

This mirror leads to your freedom, because once you understand what you're doing to keep yourself trapped, and why you're doing it, you are on the path to a beautiful life. We'll be looking into that mirror more closely in future chapters.

The second thing we'll be doing is envisioning what life will be like once you're free. Many women I've spoken with have been trapped in their prison for so long that they can't imagine any other life. They feel there's no escape. And they've given up trying. I know how it is. It's easy just to slip into survival mode and forget any other possibility exists.

But I'm here to tell you there is something better. No matter your current circumstances, there is a way out. And I'm not talking about leaving your current circumstances, though there are times when that may be necessary. What I'm talking about is crafting a new life for yourself even in the midst of where you are right now. I'm not here to help you with your marriage, your bills, or your relationships with your kids or relatives. I'm not here to promise you a bigger house or a nicer car.

What I am here to help you with is knowing you can have a better life right now. You can have the life you were meant for. You can start to dream again and live into those dreams. You can start right now to craft a much brighter future for yourself—a future where you are the one in control of your life.

"How are we going to do this?" you ask. That's what we're going to be exploring in these pages. You are going to learn how you, and you alone, are in the driver's seat of your life. Yes, circumstances happen beyond our control. But we are the ones who choose how we respond to those circumstances. We can choose in any given moment to be the victor rather than the victim. And every time we make that choice, we move ourselves one step closer to freedom.

The foundational premise of this book, and certainly a foundational premise of my life, is that I can learn to accept myself exactly as I am, who I am, where I am, right in this moment. It's amazing how much time we can spend wishing we were somewhere besides where we are right now. From that place of presence in the here and now, and from the place of loving ourselves and our life right here and now, our need to escape, to cover up, to numb out, lessens. We learn to recognize what we're doing that takes us out of that place of presence. We learn to be still and just notice what's happening on the inside.

As we are present to our emotions, our thoughts, our bodies, and every part of us, and we are loving where we are right in this moment, we can start to give ourselves permission to dream. When we've lost hope, we don't dream. Our hope is what enables us to dream.

As we continue our journey in this book, we'll talk about how it's possible to envision a bright, beautiful future for ourselves, while also loving ourselves and our life right where we are now. It sounds like a paradox that as we envision our future, we allow ourselves to be present, but that's what we're going to explore.

One primary reason we are stuck, and stay stuck, is our minds constantly create stories. The stories we keep telling ourselves fall into two categories: stories about the past, and stories about the future. Unless we are deliberate about these stories, they can leave us in a place of shame, regret, anxiety, and fear. We all carry around a lifetime of accumulated stories. And the simplest, fastest way we can break out of the negative stories that keep us in prison is to learn how to question them.

Learning to question the stories we tell ourselves goes hand in hand with the bold decision to no longer be the victim. You may have very good reasons for being a victim, and you may have had some horrific things happen to you in the past. But if you are holding this book in your hands, I have a feeling you are ready to give up your victimhood and start living the life you were meant to live. I believe you're ready to stop allowing that perpetrator to rule your life. And when I use the word "perpetrator," I'm not talking about another human being. Things have happened to you in the past. Some of those things happened to you as a result of another person's actions. But we never have to be the victim. When we relive events of the past over and over, we are being ruled by our own minds, and we are keeping ourselves in victim status. We become our own perpetrator. It's time to stop that vicious cycle.

A NEW CHAPTER

By picking up this book, you are beginning a new chapter in your life. I believe you picked it up because you are ready to take control of your life and be the victor. And I will show you how to do just that. The result is a life of gratitude and joy instead of the life you may be living right now, a life of regret, shame, fear, and despair.

And that is where the freedom lies. I've given you the bird's eye view, and now it's time to get to work.

But there are some prerequisites to getting started on this path. You may not be all in yet, and if not, that's okay. You may feel weak and shaky as you get started; this journey might feel scary, or even terrifying. But here is what you at least need to start to understand. First, you are worth it. You are worth valuing and caring for and nurturing. You are worth this journey. No matter how many different angles people, circumstances, and work are pulling on you from, you are worthy of devoting your full attention, if only for a few moments a day, to your wholeness.

Second, you are beautiful. You need to know that. We've been fed a lie about beauty in our society. You are so much more than what you look like. Your worth is not measured by any scale or tape measure. Your worth is not judged by the glamor magazine covers or the beauty pageants. We are going to discover your inner beauty, and in the process, we will start allowing that beautiful you on the inside to come out and be visible on the outside.

This may sound scary, but it's worth facing the fear, facing the shame, and facing the things that have kept you hidden away from the world so you can truly shine. It's time to really start living your life, and to be fully you, unashamedly. It's your time to shine.

QUESTIONS FOR REFLECTION

What external measures have you used to determine your worth?
_____
_____
_____
_____

Have you become your own perpetrator? Are you keeping yourself in victim status? How so?
_____
_____
_____
_____

What kind of life can you envision for yourself once you are free?
_____
_____
_____
_____

Chapter 2

Are You Hiding?

During one of my first coaching conversations with Marie, she let me know she was a loser. She told me she had never succeeded in anything. She did not see how she was going to succeed this time. All of her perceived failures added up to a huge pot of self-doubt. She just didn't think she could do it.

It didn't take too much digging for me to find out Marie had earned a bachelor's degree. Then with a little more digging, she admitted she also had a master's degree. She kept insisting the only way she had obtained these degrees was with a lot of help from her professors and advisors. Soon she reluctantly admitted to me she had also been awarded a PhD.

What? I'd never heard of someone who was just a loser obtaining a PhD. I was dumbfounded. "Did they just hand you this degree?" I asked. "Did you purchase it online for $69.95?" She laughed. She knew I was joking. "Did you cheat your way through?" I continued.

"No," she admitted. "I did the work myself. But the reason I feel I don't really deserve it is I had so much help from my advisors. Probably way more help than most people get. I can't really take credit for it."

WHAT IDENTITY ARE YOU HIDING BEHIND?

We'll come back to Marie's story in a moment, but first let me point out that every single one of us has beautiful, amazing accomplishments to celebrate. We don't have to have received a PhD or a college degree of any kind, or even a high school diploma, for that to be true. We can always find accomplishments to celebrate if we're willing to look in the mirror honestly.

And that doesn't mean we have to take all the credit for something we've done. What I reminded Marie of during our phone conversation was that an actor, leaping up onto the stage to receive his Oscar, doesn't take all the credit. He receives his award, gracefully, and proceeds to thank Mom and Dad, his best friend, his eighth-grade drama coach, his producers, his directors, and whoever else he can think of to thank.

When I tell you to take a good, hard look in the mirror, I'm asking you to start to see who you really are. Start to see past the beliefs that are holding you back and keeping you stuck. You are so much more powerful than you realize. Look back on those times when you believed you were a victim and see how you rose up and started living your life again. Begin to recognize and celebrate the strength you found inside you to put one foot in front of the other and start moving forward again.

What identity have you been hiding behind? What have you been telling yourself? *I'm a loser. I'm a failure. I'm fat. I'm lazy. I'm ugly. I'm a procrastinator.* What if I told you these are beliefs you've held onto about yourself, and the more you held onto them, the more true they became? What if there was a new angle to look at the same facts from that would allow you to come to a completely different conclusion?

But, Lynn, you protest, *I am 100 pounds overweight. I am 200 pounds overweight. I have never been called pretty in my life. I can't make myself do anything I don't want to do. I fail at everything I try. How can you tell me my beliefs aren't true?*

I am here to tell you your worth is not measured by a piece of glass in the bathroom, or by that bathroom scale, or even by a report card. Your worth is on the inside, and no one and nothing can take that away from you. We are here to uncover it, recognize it, nurture it, and tend to it, so it can shine on the outside. And the world will get to experience the beauty of you.

How are your limiting beliefs keeping you stuck? I know when I fall into the trap of thinking I'm a procrastinator, I am much more likely to procrastinate. The identity I hold onto shapes my thinking, and my thinking shapes the choices I make. When I'm clinging to self-doubt and negative beliefs, those are the beliefs I'm acting on. If I'm constantly beating myself up for being overweight, or not having any self-control, I am much more likely to turn to food to reinforce that belief and thus stay stuck in the cycle of defeat and discouragement.

I remember the day I learned how to be a procrastinator. I was at a friend's house so we could do an assignment together. We were in third grade. I was eager to get started on the project because I hadn't had a project like this in second grade. The assignment made me feel like one of the big kids. As we were about to start on it, my friend looked at me quizzically and said, "You like this, don't you?" The question caught me off guard. Yes, I did, until that moment. All of a sudden, I wasn't so sure. *Am I not supposed to like it? Is that not cool?* I asked myself. She had a cool older brother, so maybe she had picked up this attitude from him. All I know is something shifted in me that day. I didn't know what to call it, but I learned it was better to put off assignments until later. Play first, until the last minute when you know you have to get to work or risk not getting it done, and then scramble to finish on time.

I've carried that identity around with me for years—that I am a procrastinator. I don't need to remember the incident that got me started on that path to recognize this is a belief I've held onto about myself. The problem is not in the particular incident. It could have been anything, and I could have learned that coping mechanism in any number of places, or just dreamed it up myself. The problem lies in the belief.

We all create identities that feel safe to hide behind. Sometimes those identities do keep us safe, but most of the time, they just keep us playing small. Something inside of us wants more. We want to start playing a bigger game. But when we start to think there's no way out, and that we're trapped inside that identity, it can feel like a big disappointment.

So we get through life by coping. We don't get through life all at once; we have to face it one moment at a time and one day at a time. But how do we cope moment by moment when we're experiencing the pain of knowing we're not living the life we were meant to live?

WHAT ARE YOU DOING TO COPE?

What are you doing to cope with this mountain of stories, beliefs, and thoughts that have been keeping you stuck all these years? Are you turning to snack foods? Are you numbing out with sweets, desserts, and candy? Do you load up on the carbs that just keep calling your name? If you are comforting yourself with food on a regular basis, or using food to cope with stress, anger, loneliness, boredom, or whatever the emotion may be, then it's time to face it.

These are some of the hidden addictions rampant in our culture. Most of the time, for the women I work with, it's sugar and carbs. Sugar has been compared to heroin in how addictive it is. That could be overstated, but in hearing the secret pain of so many of the women I've spoken to, I'm not so sure. And when you start reading the labels on all these processed and packaged foods, you see that sugar is practically in everything. Whether it's in the form of high-fructose corn syrup, refined sugar, or any other label it's hiding under, it's everywhere.

You may have never thought of sugar, carbs, or food in general as an addiction. And that's okay if you haven't. Sugar activates the pleasure sensors in the brain in a similar way to how recreational drugs or prescription painkillers do. That didn't happen by accident. Food scientists sometimes spend their entire careers finding ways to make the processed foods we eat more addictive. The food industry doesn't *want* you only to "eat just one." If you did, business wouldn't be so great. The marketing, the packaging, the smell, look, ingredients, texture, and taste all go into that feeling of *just one more*. Irresistible is the key word. And I'd say those scientists have succeeded pretty well.

Many women struggle with prescription or recreational drugs, alcohol, and cigarettes. A lot of shame can exist around this, too, even more so than the sugar. Some of our addictions are out in the open, and some of them are hidden away. Often, even our spouse or those closest to us may not know anything is wrong.

If any of those ring true for you, I'm not bringing this up to make you feel bad. But it's crucial to your future freedom to see what may be holding you back from your transformation. When we recognize our stories are what are driving us to our addictions, it's easier to look at our addictions objectively, take a step back, and stop beating ourselves up.

Now we can just look at it. Our addictions are a cover-up for the pain we're in. Every addiction is a decision, no matter how long in the past that decision was made, to use something outside of ourselves to mask or run away from something that's happening on the inside. A big part of looking in that figurative mirror is deciding you're not going to hide from you anymore. You're not going to hide from your fears, your emotions, or your thoughts any longer.

This chapter is not about the evils of sugar, but about what we do regularly to cope with the hurt and pain we feel on the inside, and what we do to cover it up. It hardly matters in what form the cover-up comes. For me, it wasn't alcohol, drugs, or food. When I was in my mid-thirties, I retreated into a fantasy world of my own making. Looking back, I can see that was an emotional addiction.

I didn't feel I could cope with the reality of the pain I was experiencing in my marriage, and one day I allowed my mind to wander to an imaginary world of having the affection and care of another man. It felt good in the moment, and my immediate thought was, *No one will ever know. I can think whatever I want in my own mind, and it will just be my own private thoughts.*

I remember the moment so well. We were coming home from church in our minivan, kids buckled into the back two rows of seats, driving up the steep narrow road to our home in the mountains. Life should have been perfect, and on the surface, it looked like it was. But the reality was far from it.

Sitting there in the passenger seat, I was looking for relief from the pain I was living in. *No one will ever know what's going on in my mind*, I repeated to myself. *No one will ever find out.* I justified, and I retreated into a world of my own making. I thought it was only for a moment, but the flood of emotion that washed over me was so powerful in that moment that I didn't want to leave that place. It was every bit the relief I sought. It brought me comfort and a little bit of happiness. Soon, I found I was turning to that imaginary world I had created again and again. It didn't take long before I realized I was caught in a trap I was powerless to escape.

I didn't understand that day driving home the powerful hold these idle thoughts would have on me. The emotions grabbed hold of me tightly and didn't let go. Soon, I was using the thought world I had created to get through each day. I used it to give myself the energy I needed to do the next thing. I used it to rescue myself out of the mundane, but primarily out of my pain. It wasn't long, though, before I realized this was not freedom. This was a prison—a prison of my own making. What started out as a diversion, a little escape from reality, became a dungeon for me. And dungeons aren't pretty.

I eventually realized I was existing in two realities, and I was not present in either one. I had always considered myself to be a self-controlled and disciplined person. But the stark realization that I finally came to was that I was neither. I was trapped. I was stuck. And like being caught in quicksand, the more I struggled to break free, the deeper I sank. But I'd had enough, and I knew it. I wanted out.

Many of the women who sign up for a call with me are in this very place. They recognize they've had enough of the sugar and carb addictions, the eating to quell the hurt and stress in their lives, the habitual snacking in front of the TV, or whatever form it takes for them. They've had enough, and they're ready to be set free.

I finally, reluctantly, came to the unpleasant conclusion that I needed help. This realization was extremely humbling for me because I had always kept up the image, or thought I did anyway, of having it all together. I didn't like being so vulnerable and allowing my weakness to show. The thought of allowing someone in to see the chink in my armor terrified me. After struggling on my own for some time and feeling miserable, I finally turned to a friend for help. That was one of the hardest things I ever did in my entire life. I had to admit my helplessness. But I knew I had no other option.

Who could I possibly let into my inner world, who was close, but not close enough to my daily life that it wouldn't cause more harm than good? And who could I trust enough to let in on this deep secret I was harboring?

After some thought, I realized I did have a dear friend who checked all those boxes. It took me some time, but I finally picked up the phone and dialed her number. I remember that conversation well. I stammeringly blurted out the words. I was caught. I was trapped. I couldn't get out. I told her everything she needed to know and prayed she would know how to help me. It was painful because she had believed the persona I had always presented to the world—someone who had it all together. Her first words to me were merciful. *You're human. You're human.* I felt the relief flood my body. She didn't condemn me. She didn't write me off. And she didn't shame me or lecture me. *You're human.*

The next thing she told me was even more reassuring. She had struggled in the very same way I was now struggling, and she had found her way out. The funny thing is, as I look back on it, a fantasy world is not an unusual place to retreat to for women. I was not alone. And after I talked to my friend, I knew I was on my way out.

If you are struggling with addiction of any kind, a prison you can't escape from, I want you to know there is hope. And the other thing I want you to know is freedom feels so good.

It's hard for me to go back in time and reexperience my prison. I didn't know if I would have the strength to continue on or face life without the rush of those emotions carrying me through. Whatever your addiction is, whether a chemical substance or any kind of habit you can't break, you can know right now that there is life on the other side.

I struggled for about a year before reaching out to my friend for help. I ended up creating a support system around myself because I felt I was so needy that I shouldn't lean too hard on any one person. It was never easy sharing my struggle, but the three friends I ended up bringing into my support circle became my strength and gave me the ability to keep moving forward, one step at a time.

FIRST STEPS TO FREEDOM

The first step in freeing ourselves from addiction of any kind is to admit to ourselves that we have a problem. That's not always easy to do; in fact, it can be very painful. But freedom exists even in that one small step. Many of the women I talk to each week are really good at hiding themselves from the reality of their addiction.

They've been trapped for so long that the only way they can get through each day is to live in denial. Don't look in the mirror. Don't step on the scale. Don't visit with friends you haven't seen in a long time, because you realize you will be seeing a reflection of yourself in the surprised look they give you when they see all the weight you've gained.

I've spoken with women who always want to make sure they are the one taking the picture. If they show up in a picture, they don't want to see it because then they have to face what they've been attempting to hide from themselves.

Whenever a woman tells me this, it reminds me of one of my college roommates. When she received a bill or a grade report in the mail, she would quickly hide it behind her back, unopened, and carefully walk backward toward a drawer in the kitchen. With both hands behind her back, facing away from the drawer, she would open the drawer and stuff the bill inside. This wasn't easy because the drawer was already stuffed full of bills and other bits of unwanted information. But she would manage to close the drawer, still facing away from it, without ever seeing any of the contents. And then she could go happily on with her day.

I'm not sure what caused her coping mechanism of denial to be so overt, or why she took such extreme measures to avoid facing reality. But I do know she failed the one class I was taking with her because she never showed up. Whatever it was, she wasn't ready or willing to talk about it. She was hiding from herself.

What have you been doing to hide from your reality? And what is it that's causing you to hide?

When I look back on my addiction, I can see the biggest thing I was feeling was shame. My shame was so big that the thought of being exposed terrified me. Shame thrives in secrecy. Others may shame us, but they don't have the power to hold us in shame. Shame only happens when we pick it up and put it on ourselves. We have to internalize it for it to have any power over us. Others can speak shaming words over us or treat us in a way that leads us toward shame, but they can't put us in shame. That is for us to do, ourselves. Shame causes us to hide ourselves away from the outside world. It closes us in on ourselves, sometimes to the point where all we know is shame.

HIDING BEHIND SHAME

Shame. There is so much packed into those five letters. The weight of shame can be crippling, to the point where we feel as though there is no way out. Shame does have its place, though, as a way of creating social norms of behavior, such as putting on clothes before going outside. I'm not talking about shame at that level. I'm talking about the shame that keeps us hiding, playing small, not wanting to be seen.

What is shame exactly, and why do we live there?

Shame is what we feel when we are laughed at or ridiculed. More often than not, we can be living in shame, spending years of our lives there without even realizing shame is our address. We start to feel like we deserve to live there, and shame becomes not only our address, but our identity.

Children can quickly become masters of shame. We so want to fit in and be one of the crowd, and we become afraid of standing out in a negative way. If we say the wrong thing or do the wrong thing, soon we will be singled out and become the subject of the merciless ridicule that only children can deliver.

And it's not their fault. They are only picking up the behavior they've seen modeled around them. They're treating others the way they've been treated. And when I say only children can deliver shame, I mean exactly that. Adults who live in that space of shaming others to feel better about themselves are still behaving as children. They have not grown up.

It's not our job to tell them, of course, and it wouldn't do any good even if we did. But as we face our own shame, remembering that shame is delivered by children, or by adults behaving as children, can make us feel a bit better.

It's not about you. When somebody insults you, ridicules you, or somehow sets out to make you feel less than, it is not about you. In fact, it has nothing to do with you.

Let that sink in for a moment. All this time you've been thinking it's about you. You took it in; you internalized it. You can forgive yourself for that right now because you didn't know any better. Whether you consciously thought it, or gradually let the thinking take over, you adopted a story you thought was about you.

YOU THOUGHT IT WAS ABOUT YOU

You thought it was about you. What do I mean by that? The way we interact with others and the way we treat each other has, for the most part, been conditioned in us from a young age. We see certain behavior patterns in others, and without even realizing it, we treat those people in exactly the same way we've been conditioned to. We may see someone who dresses a certain way, looks a certain way, or behaves a certain way, and we react accordingly. But this reaction has nothing to do with the other person. It only has to do with what's inside of us.

Being admitted into nursing school in my early fifties was exciting and terrifying at the same time. It was terrifying, for one, because I didn't know how I was going to handle the time commitment. I was this newly single mom, working full-time at a low-paying job, trying to make ends meet so I could provide a good life for my two teenage sons. I was overseeing their home study curriculum and helping them adjust to their new life while I was adjusting to my new life as a single parent. My previous college degree, earned many years prior, was in English. I had considered healthcare-related fields as a young adult entering college, but I had this limiting belief that I was bad in math and science. This belief had held me back in school for so many years that I gravitated toward the thing I excelled in, which was anything to do with language arts.

Going to school in a math- and science-related field was brand-new territory for me. The only reason I even considered it possible was I had spent the previous twenty years homeschooling my six kids. In the process, not only did I become good at math, but I also realized I could read a textbook and understand what it was saying with the best of them. I had years of experience of my children bringing their high school textbooks to me and asking me to explain a paragraph. I could take that paragraph and break it down into its simplest form to help my child understand the concept behind it. As I was toying with the idea of going to nursing school and becoming a nurse in my fifties, I realized that if I could do that for my kids, I could do it for myself also.

I found that although nursing school was challenging, and juggling school, work, and home responsibilities took a lot of intention, for me the most difficult parts of nursing school were the hands-on skills and the interpersonal interaction.

I'm not here to talk about nursing school, per se, but the phenomenon of being thrust back into a classroom setting after almost thirty years spent more or less in my comfort zone.

All the old insecurities, the shyness and timidity, the feeling of invisibility, the feeling of being excluded, all came flooding back to me. Along with that, all the behaviors I had rarely even seen in myself, having been out of that setting for so long, were staring me straight in the face yet again.

All of a sudden, I was that shy, timid little wallflower. Except this time, I was about the oldest one in the class.

One day, I realized something. These people didn't know me from anyone. No one sent the memo to them to treat me the way I had been treated in elementary school, junior high, or high school. No one told them I was not one of the popular kids. No one told them to overlook me or not pay any attention to me. I was just another member of the class in a sea of faces.

I was the smart one, or one of the smart ones. I was the one who hung back and only spoke if called upon. Suddenly, I realized no one had put that identity on me except myself. We were all smart and highly motivated. That was how we all got into a program that only admitted forty out of 400 applicants.

My big revelation was that all of this came from inside me, and I was projecting it into the outer world. I was inviting the way I was being treated. And it's not that I was ever bullied or treated badly; I just didn't feel like I fit in. I was on the outside looking in. The cool kids were getting together to study and socialize, and I wasn't one of the cool kids. Nobody had to send out the memo informing them I was not one of the cool kids; I was the one who projected that information out into the class.

Looking back, I have to laugh. I escaped from nursing school unscathed, diploma in hand. That was all that mattered. If I had listed out my goals for my nursing school experience, being included, being one of the popular kids would not have made the list. I got the job done, I grew as a human being, and I even enjoyed much of the experience. If it had been my goal to fit in, that's where I would have put my attention. But my goal was to master the skills and learn the academic side of it well enough to rock the NCLEX exam and, more importantly, to be a competent and caring nurse.

I did that. And I'm proud of it. My point in sharing this story is that what I receive from others is a reflection of what I'm projecting out to them. I was the one who carried that junior-high identity into nursing school forty years later.

I love what that taught me because I don't think I could have learned it any other way than seeing it with my own eyes.

The point is we carry our shame around with us; we project it out into the world, and we are treated accordingly. If we project love, joy, compassion for others, gratitude, and any number of other traits, that's what we get back. Not because others have changed, but because we have changed. We are living in a new identity, and that new identity is what we are now expecting of ourselves. As we live in that new identity, our need for acceptance, approval, and appreciation lessens.

We don't really even notice how others are treating us because we are more focused on what their needs might be and how we might be able to serve them. Living in joy and gratitude makes us attractive people. Being interested in others and learning how to listen draws others to us like a magnet. When we are in our own head, wondering, *Do they like me? Am I going to say the right thing? What happens if I mess up? What happens if I make a fool of myself? Is anyone going to want to talk to me?* we are all the more likely to be overlooked.

Then we think to ourselves, *There must be something wrong with me. Why don't they like me? Why am I always on the sidelines?*

It's a self-fulfilling prophecy. But it's one that can be broken, and that's what we're setting out to do here.

What does shame do to us? It makes us afraid to step out and try lest we fail once again. We reason, *If I mess up, I will have even more to add to my list of things to be ashamed of. I'll be adding to my long list of failures, and I don't know if I can handle that. I might be publicly ridiculed. My friends and family might be ashamed of me. I will be humiliated. They'll think, "There she goes again, thinking she was competent, thinking she could do it. What a joke."*

But what if, all along, it wasn't that we were incompetent? What if it was just that we were living in an endless cycle of self-fulfilling prophecies? We live in the shame of past failures; we muster up all our courage, and we try once again in spite of believing we will never make it. We set a big lofty goal for ourselves of losing 100 pounds or working out for an hour a day, or whatever the case may be, but we only end up discouraged, defeated, and disappointed.

I just wasn't meant to succeed. All I've done my whole life is fail, so why should I even try? I might as well just give up.

But then you look at the steady weight gain, the decreasing mobility, the food cravings that just won't leave you alone, and your doctor's words echoing in your ears, *Diabetes, heart disease, or stroke are just around the corner if you don't do something now.*

And all you can say in response is, *I'll do better tomorrow.*

The reason you don't do better tomorrow—or even if you do, it doesn't last—is you haven't learned how to break out of the cycle keeping you stuck.

Marie was experiencing shame in her inability to take credit for her accomplishments. She had already written the story that she was a loser; that she needed help to get her degrees only reinforced that previously held belief. So she completely missed the acknowledgment of all the hard work, perseverance, intelligence, and everything else that could have only come from the inside. Her beliefs kept her from stepping into the greatness that was already there within herself.

HIDING BEHIND GUILT

We can hide behind guilt. Guilt can bring us to a place of self-loathing when we allow it to master us. When we are consumed by guilt, it means we haven't forgiven ourselves. The pain of guilt can be so great that it causes us to dive deeper into whatever the addiction is that's keeping us from facing our pain.

What's the difference between guilt and shame? It's not my place, nor my purpose, to go into the minute distinctions between these terms. But we can be filled with shame just for existing in this world. It encompasses our feelings that we're just not enough. We don't measure up. We're too short or too tall, too fat or too thin. We're not pretty enough, smart enough, athletic enough, graceful enough. Whatever it is, we don't have it, and we feel shame.

On the other hand, we feel guilt over things we did or didn't do. We didn't keep our commitment or our word. We let someone down. We cheated on a test. We covered up a mistake we should have admitted to. I could go on and on. These are the things we like to put out of our minds. But the problem is we can't really do that. We can ignore it and hide the unpleasant truth away from ourselves. We can cover it up, and we can justify it.

Guilt isn't a pleasant topic to address. And facing it can be downright terrifying. It's one of the big reasons for addiction because all of our addictions stem from a desire to escape the pain we're feeling. We don't want to feel it because it doesn't feel good, so we turn to the alcohol, the food, the romance novels, or the fantasy world.

It doesn't do any good when others tell us, "Hey, don't worry about it." That does nothing to take away our guilty feelings.

Unforgiveness and guilt are close cousins. When we are living in guilt, it means we have not received forgiveness for ourselves. And when we are living in unforgiveness, we are caught in a prison of depending on someone else's behavior to be free. Unforgiveness rarely hurts the other party as much as it hurts us as the one harboring the unforgiveness. When we harbor anger and resentment against another person, it can eat us alive. It doesn't hurt the other person nearly as much as it hurts us.

Unforgiveness is an open wound that, if allowed to fester, will infect us with bitterness. Bitterness is a poison to our soul. It steals our joy, takes away our gratitude, and locks us into a deep, dark dungeon. We often hang onto that unforgiveness because we believe the person who did us wrong does not deserve to be forgiven. But when we think like that, we only harm ourselves.

The truth is you deserve to be freed from this prison because you are a woman of tremendous worth. Even if you can't see your way toward forgiving the one who did the wrong, you owe it to yourself to forgive. I've heard it said that unforgiveness is like drinking poison and expecting the other person to get sick. That's what we are doing to ourselves when we don't forgive.

HIDING BEHIND OUR VICTIM STATUS

Another place we can hide in is our victim status. Life has dealt us an unfair hand, and we are the innocent victim. Often, I see this status manifesting as martyrdom. I'm giving my life for everyone else, and that's just the way it is. I am needed; nothing will get done without me, so I must sacrifice myself on behalf of others. We see this as noble and heroic. But when we can start to see it as self-serving, we can start to find our way out of it. I'm not saying it's wrong to serve others or to give up things we would enjoy in favor of others having a better life, but when this behavior manifests as playing the victim or the martyr, it's unhealthy and never really benefits the recipient.

I know I used to fit into several of these categories in my prison of addiction, but the hardest one to consciously give up was my reputation. My first husband and I thought we had a reputation to uphold because we were in Christian ministry, so even though I knew better, it was really hard to admit that what appeared on the outside didn't match what was on the inside. I found it so liberating to confide in my friend. On my road to true freedom, I found I no longer needed to hide. I enjoyed my newfound transparency. I no longer needed to pretend to be something or someone I wasn't. I could finally start learning how to be me.

If you are hiding behind the façade of perfectionism or just wanting everyone to think you've got it all together, I can tell you with 100 percent confidence that it is so much better to be free. As you set out on this journey toward freedom, toward letting the bright daylight shine into all the dark corners of your life, you will start to breathe easier and feel lighter. As you look back at your old life of hiding behind shame, guilt, unforgiveness, reputation, or any of the other places you hide, I'm here to ask you: Are you ready to give it all up and step into the beautiful sunlight of freedom? If so, keep reading because it's coming.

QUESTIONS FOR REFLECTION

What accomplishments can you celebrate? What are you proud of?

_____
_____
_____
_____
_____

What are some limiting beliefs you've been hanging onto?

_____
_____
_____
_____
_____

How are these limiting beliefs contributing to keeping you stuck?

_____
_____
_____
_____
_____

How have you internalized the shame others have sent your way? How has shame held you back?

_____
_____
_____
_____
_____

What have you been doing to hide from your reality?

___

What will freedom look like for you?

___

Chapter 3

Daring to Hope Again

Our next step toward true freedom is to realize that yes, something better is out there for you.

When I first began a coaching relationship with Linda, she was deep in simultaneous despair and terror. She felt both she and others had ruined her life beyond repair, and she was living in a constant state of hopelessness. Most of our early conversations were spent in her sobbing. She had lived in turmoil for so long that she could barely think, let alone function.

Her current situation wasn't all that terrified her. She had lived in a constant state of chaos and panic for as long as she could remember.

I want to make it clear here that I am not a counselor or therapist. We don't need to go deep into the past. As a coach, I help women look at where they are now and decide what path they want to be on. Part of this process involves taking a look at what we believe about our life right now. As we do that, we can start to see it's not about what other people have done to us, and it's not about all the mistakes we've made. Instead, it's our beliefs about those events that shape our current state of mind.

Even the most traumatic and scary events can be tamed in our minds as we realize nothing truly happens to us. Everything happens for us, no matter the intent of any other person.

I know it can be hard to imagine this when someone is standing over you screaming that he is going to kill you while he proceeds to break your bones.

I'm not telling you this means we have to sit passively while someone is committing crimes against us. And it doesn't mean if we believe we're destitute, we don't make a plan.

The truth is that when we can embrace our current reality and know we are okay right in this moment, our mind clears, and we are then free to plan and take the very next possible right action.

I watched this time and time again during my sessions with Linda. Each time, she was able to lift herself out of her current turmoil and find the peace and presence of mind available to her in that moment. Even though she still didn't see the way out, she was able to find enough peace in that moment to take the next step forward. She started being able to make decisions from a place of peace and security instead of panic and terror. Almost in spite of herself, she watched her relationships with her children and her brother improve. She saw her dating life improve dramatically as she took each next step.

At first, Linda didn't see how she would be able to eat or even have a roof over her head. She could have made so many bad choices out of desperation. Now she is in a stable, secure, abundant relationship. She knows she never would have reached this situation if she hadn't taken the steps I brought her through.

Just like I'm not a therapist or counselor, I'm not specifically a relationship coach. But it is an unexpected delight for me to see my clients' relationships improve right along with their health and food choices.

Linda credits me with saving her life. I have no idea where she would be right now if she hadn't booked that first call with me and committed to finding a new life for herself. I'm so grateful to have had the opportunity to bring this beautiful woman into a place of peace and freedom.

IS THERE LIFE AFTER ADDICTION?

When I was caught in my web of emotional addiction, I knew I wanted to be free. But a scary thought lurked in the back of my mind: What if I could never be happy again? What if the fantasy world I had retreated into was my only source of happy emotions? What if all I had to look forward to, if I gave up this fantasy world, was a bleak, monotone existence?

Now I'm the one telling my clients there is life beyond dessert. Once, when I made an offhand remark one evening in one of our group coaching sessions, my client Judy fixated on it for the rest of the session. "Never eat a Christmas cookie again?" she said. "Won't my life just be miserable if I can never, ever again eat a Christmas cookie?"

If you've never been addicted to sugar, maybe this thought seems silly to you. But when she raised that concern, I could instantly relate. I've had those thoughts about food, but even more so about that emotional addiction I was caught in. It doesn't really matter how foolish that thought seems to someone on the outside. When you are struggling with addiction, that thought is very real.

But you weren't meant to be a slave to anything. You were meant to be free. I experienced an emotional rush in the fantasy world I was living in. We experience a sugar high when we indulge in some decadent dessert. We can use sugar, emotions, alcohol, or prescription drugs as an escape from real life. Believe it or not, Linda used chaos and confusion as coping mechanisms to get herself through each day. But you were meant to live your life, not retreat from it. There is so much more. Many of us zone out into the black hole of YouTube videos, Netflix, or TV. Others do it through romance novels or magazines. It doesn't matter what you use to escape from life, it is still just an escape. You were meant for more. Are you ready to start living your life?

You can start by imagining what freedom really looks like. As was the case with me, this may seem scary. Can I really go on living without this crutch I've depended on for so long?

Many women I talk to have been locked in their prison for so long they can't imagine what freedom looks like. Life has become a continuous cycle of resolving to do better, actually doing better for a couple of hours or a couple of days or a couple of weeks, growing weary, slipping back into apathy, giving in to the old habits, and then beating themselves up for having done so. They will stay in that state of shame, guilt, and remorse for some time. Eventually, when the latest incident has faded far enough from their memory so as not to be quite so painful, they will pick themselves back up and start the whole cycle again.

Why is it that our resolve doesn't last? How do we slip so easily back into our old ways even as we loathe ourselves for doing so?

I want to say it again: You were meant for more. Motivation and willpower are never there when you need them. We need something that will override those ideas, that will lift us up above all the old ways that haven't worked.

LEARNING TO DREAM AGAIN

As humans, we have the ability to dream. It's one of those things that makes us human. But it's one of those things that vanishes when life gets hard. We get discouraged, and we slip into fear and defeat.

A lot of our depression comes from simply giving up hope. Hope is our ability to dream of a bigger and better future for ourselves. That's one reason I start with dreaming in my work with my clients. I tell them it's time to start dreaming again. Most of them have a really hard time with that, but as we keep working on it, it gets easier.

That's where I went the other day with my client Kathy. We pinpointed that her fear of disappointment, her fear of failing yet again, and the very real chronic pain she lives with were keeping her stuck and unable to dream of a higher fitness level for herself.

"What if your pain were gone?" I asked her. "What if you knew you couldn't fail? Take pain and fear off the table. What would it look like?" She didn't know.

"That's okay," I reassured her. "There is no shame in not knowing. All I want you to do is open yourself up to the possibility that there could be more for you in your future. What would it look like? What would light you up?"

After some thought, she recognized the ability to run again, pain free, would ignite that spark. I could hear it in her voice as she spoke the words.

That was a place to start. I was thrilled for her. We can't get anywhere if all we see is hopelessness. We need that little spark that we can fan into a flame. Now we can start working on what it will take to get there. "I can't" becomes "How can I?" Curiosity replaces fear.

It was a very bleak, dark time in my life when I lost the ability to dream. I honestly just wanted to die. My life appeared so hopeless. I wasn't going to take myself out, but I was definitely wishing it would happen, and happen soon. I just couldn't imagine a future for myself that I wanted to be in. I couldn't see beyond the darkness and pain I was living in every day. And death seemed like the easy way out.

As I write these words, those days seem so distant. I'm dreaming again. I'm living into the beautiful future I have envisioned for myself. And that doesn't mean I'm not content now as I dream of things in the future that will really light me up. I'm full of gratitude for this beautiful life I've been granted. We can live in the present, live in contentment and gratitude and abundance, and still dream of an even brighter future for ourselves. It's not only okay; I would say it's vital. And it's so rare.

Very few people ever write down or speak of a vision for their life, let alone articulate goals and steps they can take to reach their vision and bring that dream to fruition.

Why? Just like Kathy, we become locked in by fear. Fear of pain, fear of disappointment, fear of shame. Others have watched us try and fail so many times that when we start on a new diet plan, they just roll their eyes. Then they sit back and watch us fall flat on our face once again. *See, I told you so.* We pick ourselves back up and try again, but this time we are quieter about it. We've learned to keep it to ourselves. Our hope and our dream begin to fade and die. We wonder if we should just give up.

Are you ready to free yourself from that prison of fear and shame and start really living your life? Are you ready to start dreaming again?

What lights you up? Maybe it's the ability to travel. Maybe it's not only keeping up with family on a mountain hiking trail but even leading the way. Maybe it's just feeling great in your own skin, walking down the beach with the sand between your toes and experiencing the thrill of being alive. Maybe it's being able to go out with friends and not worry about them thinking you put on a few more pounds since the last time they saw you. In fact, they're surprised at how great you look. Maybe it's being able to go out dancing with your partner, knowing you look fabulous and you're rocking the dance floor.

Whatever it is, think about what would really light you up, and take impossibility off the table. What would really do it for you? Can you dare to write it down? Can you dare to allow yourself to really feel it? Can you dare to hope again?

Once you've dreamed it, I want you to know you can achieve it. But it starts with the dream. It starts with allowing that dream to light you up. When you allow yourself to breathe in that vision, it interrupts the endless cycle in your brain that's telling you that you'll never measure up.

Most of us have been trying to whip ourselves into shape. If we could only find the right self-deprecating words to beat ourselves up with and make ourselves feel really awful about where we are right now, we might finally be able to get back on track. But that is the opposite of what this sort of behavior will really do for us. We will never get there by living in negativity. We need a spark of inspiration and hope to break out of that old cycle and get ourselves moving forward again.

It starts with the dream. The dream sparks hope. We start to feel it, and that beautiful future that we are envisioning for ourselves starts coming into sharper focus. We start valuing ourselves enough to allow ourselves to dream. The vision starts driving us. As we live more and more into that vision, we stop allowing those little villains of shame and guilt and all the rest to drive the car. Self-loathing, depression, guilt, and shame start taking the backseat in our lives. We stop feeding them and they become smaller and quieter. They kick at the seat in front of them less and less. Pretty soon, we start wondering why we put up with them for so long. We start to live again.

ENVISIONING A BRIGHT FUTURE

Few of us are naturally good at envisioning a beautiful future for ourselves. Most of us have to work at this ability. Maybe when we were kids we could do it, but somewhere along the line, we lost that gift of imagination. It's not actually lost. It just went into hiding. Can you remember when you used to dream? What did you dream of?

We can all visualize far more easily and readily than we think we can. How do I know this? Every time we worry, every time we become gripped with fear or panic, it's because we have envisioned something in our future that we don't want to have happen. Yes, it's true. We're able to visualize so vividly that our heart rate goes up. Our mouth goes dry. Our stomach is tied up in knots. In living color, we watch our worst fears being played out, and we experience it as if it were really happening.

That's the scary future we *don't* want to have happen. But it has been played out so many times in our minds that when the time comes, it's the reality our subconscious mind gravitates toward. It becomes a self-fulfilling prophecy. We are on autopilot, driving headlong toward the unpleasant or disastrous future. *See, I knew it. Nothing good ever happens to me.*

That was the type of future Linda was living into. I still help pull her back out of it from time to time. I remind her that her future is bright and beautiful. She doesn't have to live in fear any longer.

How do we start dreaming, in the happy dream sense, once again? The kind of dream that when we wake up, we want to finish it because it was so pleasant? I'm not really talking about the sleepy kinds of dreams. I'm talking about the wide-awake kind—the kind where you get to choose how it plays out. The daydreaming kind. I'm amazed at how rare it is for women over fifty, at least the ones I talk to, to dream. They've forgotten how. They've given up hope of things ever being better. It's a big part of my job in my work with clients to keep on encouraging them to dream. It's so foundational to making real progress in changing their lives that even when they've come up with a dream, I need to encourage them to bring it to the forefront of their minds. I find that it slips away and is easily forgotten. And that's because it's a new thought pattern. It's not the frequency our minds have been living in. It takes some work, but it's enjoyable work.

We need to see it clearly. Having tabs up on our computer of exotic places we want to travel to, or outdoor activities or adventures that we want to participate in, can help make the picture clearer. We can make a dream board or vision board with printed-out versions of our dream destinations or some representation of what we want to accomplish. It could be clothes we want to be able to wear, or a new dance step we want to learn. There is no right or wrong answer here. It's whatever lights you up. A vision board just makes it a little more real. And when you put it up on the wall next to your bed, or in the bathroom, or wherever you'll see it frequently, you'll remember to hold that vision of the beautiful, joyful life you want for yourself.

DREAMING IT UNTIL YOU FEEL IT

After we can see it, we need to feel it. This is known as emotionalizing. Just as when you imagine your worst-case scenario, and your stomach gets tied up in knots, now you are going to imagine your dream so vividly that it makes your heart sing. Yes, that means you need to believe it's possible. But if you can believe all your scary visions of your future, what is stopping you from really living into the best case? Self-help author Napoleon Hill said, "Whatever the mind can conceive and believe, you can achieve." What's holding you back?

You may be wondering, at this point, why this ability to dream, and see and feel your dream vividly, is so important. Have you ever bought a car that you thought was unique in some way, but after you drove it off the lot, you started seeing it everywhere? That happens because you're now tuned into that car. The thing is, our brains block millions of pieces of data from our conscious minds every day. Our conscious minds can't take in every bit of information because there's just too much of it. Our brain has a way of becoming highly selective about what it brings to our conscious awareness. Otherwise, we would go crazy and have no room for the important stuff.

But we can consciously choose what we turn our attention to. We have a choice in the matter. And what we choose to focus on is what usually ends up manifesting in our lives, for better or worse. I'm not talking about the Law of Attraction. All I'm saying is we naturally gravitate toward what we're focused on. Both our unconscious and conscious choices keep drawing us closer. We notice opportunities we didn't notice before. We are drawn in the direction of our dreams.

Have you ever decided you were going to cut back on calories, only to find that suddenly the most decadent, tempting foods were everywhere? That's because you were focusing on all the foods you *couldn't* have. You wanted to cut calories, but to do that, you had to become hyper-focused on the food. That led to not being able to get it out of your mind. And then chances are, sooner or later, you gave into temptation and scarfed down that one last piece of birthday cake that was calling your name. Calories be damned. At least now you could have some peace. That's a big reason why diets, for most of us, are destined to fail. You're putting your focus in the wrong place.

What if, instead, you pictured yourself walking down the beach, sand between your toes, looking great and feeling even better? You can add whatever details you want to that image or come up with your own. When you can feel the surf splashing over your feet as you walk along, and you can hear the seagulls, and most of all you feel your heart welling up with joy and gratitude that you've come so far and accomplished so much to get to this place—that changes something inside your psyche. When you bring yourself back to the here and now, you look at that piece of cake differently. You ask yourself, "Is it really that important? Do I need it? Or is it one more little thing that's standing in the way of the life I really want for myself?"

Suddenly, it's not "oh, so hard" to make the right choices for yourself because that dream is so real you can hear the surf rushing up the sandy beach. You may be thinking, "Yes, but I can resist everything but temptation." I am here to tell you the reason you can't resist the temptation is because that's how you've trained yourself for decades. You can retrain your brain.

I'm not saying this to be insulting. We all fall into this trap in one way or another. But it's the child brain that "wants it and wants it now." It's an adult characteristic to be able to delay gratification and choose something we want more than the immediate, momentary pleasure. We don't have to be the toddler throwing the temper tantrum in the middle of the grocery store aisle. We can build a new set of responses based on a new set of beliefs and a new set of dreams of the life we really want for ourselves.

And that all begins, oddly enough, with a deliberate decision to love and accept ourselves exactly as we are, where we are, right now in this moment.

QUESTIONS FOR REFLECTION

Is something holding you back from dreaming? What is it?
_____
_____
_____
_____

What would light you up? What did you dream about when you were younger?
_____
_____
_____
_____

Are you in the habit of envisioning a scary or unpleasant future for yourself (i.e., worrying)? Can you shift that image to a bright, beautiful future? What does that future look like for you?
_____
_____
_____
_____

Chapter 4

Accepting Where We Are Right Now

In my early forties, I enjoyed a high level of fitness. I didn't get there overnight, of course. Up until my late thirties, I had spent most of the previous sixteen years either pregnant with one of my six kids or nursing, with only brief intervals of being or doing neither. I look back on that time with gratitude and loads of fond memories, so I'm not complaining. But when the youngest of the six was old enough to be left in the care of the older kids, I started thinking about getting outside all by myself. That had rarely happened in the previous sixteen years.

We lived in an amazing spot. It was my dream home and my dream location. Every once in a while, since we had moved from the suburbs of Boise, Idaho, into the mountains, I would have the fleeting thought that these miles of dirt roads in the beautiful surroundings would have been my dream come true as a runner in my teens. Back then, I'd had visions of becoming a decent endurance runner. But both in high school and college, I was plagued with shin splints, which I was later told were caused by my bones growing so fast that the muscles didn't have time to catch up. In any event, the shin splints were excruciatingly painful, and after two major bouts with them in high school and college, I ended my thoughts of being a real runner.

But while living in Pullman, Washington, in my later college years, I discovered that dirt roads were the antidote to shin splints, as was easing up on the pressure on myself to perform. I learned that running just for fun on the soft dirt roads was empowering and exhilarating. That was short-lived, though, because at that time, I was newly married and pregnant with our first child.

The story picks up sixteen years later in my late thirties. I assumed I was too old to run. After all, I had never heard of anyone in their late thirties who was a runner. That was just not part of my world. But the thought did cross my mind that those dirt roads all around us would have been pure heaven, if only I weren't so old.

All that is to say I had no expectations on myself as I first ventured outside to go for short, solitary morning walks. It felt glorious being alone in the silence in the beautiful mountain surroundings. I was just glad to be outside without having to carry or coax along little ones or find ways to make it an educational experience for the older ones.

I won't go into it all here because that is not the point of the story. But I actually did get in shape, start running, and become pretty good at it, too. That was one of the greatest joys of my life, to be at that level of fitness. I built up my strength and endurance, along with my mental stamina, over a number of years up until my mid-forties. My love of the sport, the dirt roads, and the massive hills led to my success. I went so much farther than I had ever dreamed possible.

I tell you that as a contrast to what came next. Life became stressful. My running became more infrequent. I started having a health issue

I had dealt with during pregnancy that really slowed me down. I gained five pounds. My marriage was going downhill. My mom fell ill with pancreatic cancer, and I stayed at her bedside for about five weeks before she passed away. On came another five pounds. I separated from my husband of almost thirty years and got an apartment right next to the freeway. It was a far cry from the wonderland I had known for the previous twenty years. I brought my two youngest sons to live with me in the apartment. Suddenly, I was a single mom working a full-time, low-paying job, going to school in hopes of getting into nursing school, and trying to provide a stable home environment for my two boys, who were fourteen and seventeen at the time.

As I worked my way through nursing school, any thought of my previous levels of fitness had long since fallen by the wayside. Nursing school was a lot tougher than I had imagined it would be. I was still working thirty hours a week during that time. And yes, the weight kept creeping on. I was 100 percent in survival mode. I knew I had to succeed at nursing school. Failure was not an option.

Even though I already had earned a degree a few decades earlier, that time of my life stretched me beyond anything I had experienced previously. Eventually, though, the pressure let up. I graduated from nursing school and started my new life as a registered nurse. I started thinking about running again. But thinking about it is a lot different than actually doing it. I was a good twenty-five to thirty pounds heavier than when I had been a runner a decade previously. The memory was still fresh of being in really great shape for a forty-something female. Now I was postmenopausal and heavier than I had ever been, not counting pregnancy.

Where I used to feel like I was flying, it now felt more like a plod. It didn't feel good. The first time I had gotten in shape as an older adult, I had no expectations on myself. I didn't even know it was possible to get in shape at that age. And now, a decade and a half later, I knew it was possible. But that dream seemed so far away.

Finally, the realization hit me: "I can't be where I'm not. I can't go back in time and start from where I used to be. I have to start from where I am right now. And that means that I have to accept where I am right now. In other words, I need to face reality. I need to acknowledge that I weigh more than I did back then, I'm older than I was back then, and being postmenopausal, the same rules may not apply." I didn't even know what those rules were.

LEARNING SELF-ACCEPTANCE

Learning to accept ourselves exactly as we are right now can be tough. We women can be so hard on ourselves. We talk to ourselves in ways we would never talk to a friend. So many of us are filled with self-loathing and disgust as we look at our habits that are sabotaging us. We look in the mirror or we look at a photo and we look away. We can't bear to face what's before our eyes. And it doesn't matter if it's 10 pounds, 50 pounds, or 200 pounds. I've spoken with enough women to know that the self-loathing and self-criticism are the same no matter how much weight is involved. We are so good at beating ourselves up.

How do we learn to accept ourselves right where we are, right in this moment? It can seem like a big hurdle in front of us when self-criticism is all we've ever known. And for many of us, that critical nature is what we use to drive ourselves forward. We think we need to be at war with ourselves internally to make any progress.

I am reminded of when I was leaning so heavily on my friends to help me out of the prison of addiction I was in. I was so ashamed of myself, and I lived in that shame every day. After a particularly bad day, I called one of those friends. I asked her, or maybe pleaded with her would be more accurate, "Would you please knock some sense into me? Would you please beat me up a little bit?"

She only laughed and said, "I think you are doing quite a good enough job of beating yourself up. You don't need my help to do that!"

Wow. That hit me hard. I suddenly realized I was beating myself up all the time. And here I was thinking I needed more of it. This caused me to think. *Is beating myself up really what is going to save me? Or am I only digging my hole deeper as I do this?*

I have no idea how long it took me, but I do believe that one conversation with my friend started me down a new path. I started looking at what I really wanted my life to look like. I started caring for myself. It was about that time I was starting to run. I used the physical and mental stamina I was building to run up long hills to represent the inner strength I was building in overcoming my negative thought patterns. When I got to the top of the big hill, I would pump my fists in the air and celebrate. I allowed that to be a celebration of me. I was getting stronger. I was building my endurance. And it was exhilarating. I loved watching that incremental improvement. It filled me with a joy I hadn't experienced in a long time. And it was a real joy, not a rush of inflated emotions that could fade away as quickly as they came on.

I learned to capture the confidence I was building in my running and channel it into the knowledge that I could transform my inner life as well. I focused on my spiritual well-being. I learned anew what real joy and self-forgiveness felt like. I had no need to beat myself up anymore. This book is not about my spiritual journey. Someday, I might write that one for those who are interested. Suffice it to say right here, my relationship with God became more precious to me than any earthly relationship. And living in that place strengthened my other relationships.

ARE YOU BEATING YOURSELF UP?

A huge part of learning how to value yourself is learning how not to beat yourself up. That understanding can then manifest itself into creating a vision for something better. Is there anything better than a piece of cheesecake or a box of cookies? When you've discovered the joy of healthy activities, the joy of that whole world that awaits you on the other side of your addiction, you will look back on those questions and laugh. You will wonder how you could have possibly ever thought like that. *Why did dessert hold such a high place in my life? How could it have ever had such a hold on me?* That's exactly how I look back on my addiction. I still have to practice not cringing and not retreating back into shame when I think about that time in my life. But now when I remember that time, the overwhelming feeling is one of gratitude, because that time, among others, has brought me to this beautiful place in my life where I am now.

If you don't think you're hard on yourself—that you are only being honest and telling it like it is—I invite you to ask yourself the following questions: Would you ever tell your best friend, "Oh, you are so lazy!"? Would you ever tell her she is stupid and ugly? Would you ever dream that she deserves to hear such things? My guess is no. If you care about her and her feelings, you know she struggles with her own sense of self-worth. You know she needs your encouragement, not your condemnation. If she struggles with procrastination or with her weight, you understand she needs the encouragement to be lifted out of that place, and that stating to her something she already believes to be true does nothing to help her out of her stuck place.

We understand this about others, but why is it so difficult for us to bring the same uplifting, encouraging words we know our friend needs to ourselves? Why do we beat ourselves down with words we would not say to our worst enemy?

I invite you to start being your own best friend. At the very least, I invite you to stop being your own worst enemy. I invite you to end the war that is going on between your ears, one in which there is no winner.

The truth is, if you want to reach a new level of happiness and fulfillment in your life, the first step is to end that war. And the first step toward ending the war is simply to be aware of the inner critic's voice. What self-deprecating words are constantly running through your mind and beating you down? If you are not already journaling, this would be a great place to start. Get those accusations you are constantly hurling at yourself down on paper. You need to start seeing them for what they are. You need to start recognizing them when they rise to the surface of your conscious mind. Only then can you address them and put them in their place. With each one that you notice, ask yourself: *Would I say this to my best friend? Do I really believe these are the words she needs to hear? What could I say to her instead?*

Accepting yourself where you are right here in this moment does not mean stagnating or staying stuck where you are. But getting out of the hole doesn't happen by digging it deeper around yourself. You won't get out of it that way. So, let's start looking at what will lift you out of the hole, that stuck place you are in, and get you started on a new path for yourself.

LEARN TO BE YOUR OWN BEST FRIEND

It's time for you to start being your own best friend. This may not happen all in one day. I know it hasn't for me. But I can start with those things I genuinely love and appreciate about myself and start building from there. I can stop beating myself up for things beyond my control. I can look at my past accomplishments and things I am genuinely proud of in myself, and I can know if I can do that thing, then I can do the next thing too.

In fact, every single thing that's ever happened to me in my life, every experience, every word that has been spoken to me, every slight or every act of caring, has brought me to this point, here and now, in this very moment. And if I can be grateful right in this moment—and I can, no matter what, because I choose to—then I can be grateful for everything that has brought me to this moment.

If you find yourself reacting to those words, and you find the argument rising up in your own mind that there's no way you can be grateful for this thing that has happened to you, this thing that somebody did to you, then I invite you just to be still right now and open your mind to the idea that this may be the very thing that will set you free. Is it worth considering? Are *you* worth exploring this idea?

I invite you right now to step into gratitude. Gratitude can't exist in the presence of regret. Those two ideas are mutually exclusive. If we are beating ourselves up for where we are right now, it's because we're living in the regret of choices that we have made in the past. Fortunately, the opposite is also true. Regret can't exist in the presence of gratitude. When we fill our lives with gratitude, suddenly we can be content. We can accept ourselves. We can accept our circumstances and make friends with our past.

As we practice gratitude, it becomes a habit. It brings us peace. Then we can start accepting where we are right now. And it goes even further than that. We can start loving where we are right now. We can start "loving what is," as author and speaker Byron Katie says. As we start to do that, life becomes beautiful. It was beautiful all along, but we didn't have eyes to see it. We were too busy looking at all the ways we've messed up and all the things that have been done to us that have kept us being the victim.

THE WAR IS OVER

As we accept ourselves and begin to love what is, we start to experience peace. The war in our mind ends. There may still be skirmishes, and we may have to remind ourselves that the war has been won. But the war is over. Our minds become quiet. We start to experience presence.

We will talk more about presence in upcoming chapters, but right now, it is enough to know that presence of mind is a gift. It brings us to a place of quiet and calm. When we are in addiction, we are in a state of chaos. That is the opposite of presence. The state of presence is a beautiful place to live, but we so rarely find it because we are afraid of the emotions simmering within us just beneath the surface.

We're afraid of the turmoil we're currently living in. We're afraid that staring straight into the reality of our chaos and our addiction will lead us to giving up in despair. We are afraid we won't be able to face the shame that a look in the mirror will bring. But if we face into all this with the right support and the right tools, this is exactly where we can start to find hope.

Addiction happens when we are reaching out toward something outside of ourselves to soothe some emotional or mental pain we are experiencing. We are reaching to the outside to try to fix something we're experiencing on the inside. That's all that addiction is, plain and simple. I can think of a few exceptions to this, such as babies who are born addicted to meth. And while none of us choose to be addicted, we did make the choice to use some substance, thought, or action to ease the pain we were experiencing. I consciously chose the thought. And I consciously decided I would never tell anyone, and that no one would ever find out. That was how I justified it in the moment. I chose secrecy, which, of course, is the fast track to a life of shame. What I didn't choose was how that thought pattern would grab hold of me and not let go. I never dreamed on that day that I would end up trapped. And the more I struggled to break free, the more stuck I became.

Have you ever tried not to think a thought? We have probably all done that at one time or another. Maybe you thought you could escape your addiction by distracting yourself or choosing not to think about it. This, still, is not freedom. The only way to conquer addiction once and for all is to face it squarely, head on.

How do we begin to face those things ensnaring us? How do we break free? The answer lies in learning how to be present.

QUESTIONS FOR REFLECTION

Are you critical of yourself? Do you beat yourself down with words? Is there a war going on in your mind?

_____
_____
_____
_____

How can you start accepting yourself right where you are, right now?

_____
_____
_____
_____

Chapter 5

Learning to Be Present

I've already shared with you that my emotions and thoughts became quite a battleground for me. The more I focused on not thinking those thoughts, the more omnipresent they were. This was, of course, very discouraging to me. Have you ever tried not thinking a thought? Then you probably know what I mean. But as I was learning to carry forward the strength I was gaining physically and mentally with my running, I began to see some progress. I began to tell myself that if I could run up a three-mile-long hill without stopping, I could also conquer my thoughts and emotions.

In running, I found stillness. That may not make much sense since when I'm running I'm obviously moving my body, but my mind became more and more still. I could focus in on my breathing and the rhythm of my footsteps on the dirt road. My mind cleared and I started to feel free. I found a happiness I hadn't known for a long time. I became more at peace within myself.

A big realization for me was I could learn how to make friends with my emotions instead of fighting them all the time. I realized I am not my emotions. My emotions are a part of me, and they are a part of what make me human. But they are not me. They do not define me. I learned I could allow them to wash over me as a part of experiencing my humanity. I could experience them with gratitude. Gratitude for being alive, for being human. I didn't have to let them control me or control my thoughts. As I made friends with my emotions, I began to see them as separate from myself. Emotions are not good or evil all by themselves. They just are. When we interpret them in such a way that we change our thought patterns based on them, we open the door to allowing them to take control of our lives.

WHO DO I WANT TO BE?

We all make decisions based on emotion, and that's okay. In fact, it's a good thing. If we lived our lives purely by logic, our world would be robotic and flat. So what do I mean by not letting my emotions control me? I mean I get to choose the life I really want. I get to choose what I want it to look like and feel like. I get to choose joy. I get to choose what will characterize my life. In other words, I get to choose which emotions and feelings I'm going to live in.

I faced this choice in a big way during my first go-round with college (not the middle-aged college days). I was in the marching band. A guy in band named John pretty much annoyed the heck out of everyone. I'm not sure what drove him to be this way, but somehow he managed to get under everyone's skin. One day we were all walking back from our rehearsal on the football field to the band room. I don't know if John was being more obnoxious than usual, but as other band members were getting more and more fed up with him and responding accordingly, he managed to turn up the intensity of his sarcasm. I was usually pretty quiet, but for some reason, in that moment, I joined in the fray and blurted something out. I honestly don't remember what I said. It was similar to how others were interacting to John, and it was obviously how he was accustomed to being treated. He responded in kind, with the biting sarcasm he was known for.

But my response didn't sit well with me. I knew that wasn't who I was. I realized in that moment that sarcasm was the easy way out. It was easy humor, usually at somebody else's expense. I knew that wasn't how I wanted to live, or who I wanted to be known as. Not that I felt superior to anyone else; I just realized it wasn't me. In fact, I felt far from superior in that moment. I felt pretty low. I had said something mean, unkind. It didn't matter that everyone else was behaving in the same way. I regretted what I had said.

I pulled up alongside John as we walked along. I'm sure he was bracing himself for another attack.

"John, I'm sorry for what I said to you. It was wrong, and that's not how I want to treat you or anyone."

He didn't say much, if anything, beyond a casual, "Oh, that's okay." But it didn't matter. Who did I want to be? I knew right then it was a choice. I didn't have to "go with the flow." I suddenly knew I needed to live my life in sincerity and kindness, even if I was considered dull and boring. Even if it meant not being liked or approved of. That was okay with me. I needed to be true to whom I perceived myself to be on the inside.

I learned maybe a year or two later, inadvertently, that John thought highly of me. I was told he had raved about what a wonderful person he thought I was. I hadn't apologized to him so he would think well of me. I just knew I needed to speak my truth. His opinion had to have been based on that one encounter. We never know what an impact, positive or negative, our words will have on another. On that day, I had reacted based on emotion. I didn't like the reaction, so I decided on a different path for myself, and I course-corrected. We are always going to be doing that. We can make our decisions based on the emotions most congruent with the life we want. We can define ourselves based on the characteristics and emotions we choose to define ourselves by, rather than allowing our emotions to rule and define us.

EMBRACING OUR EMOTIONS

During the year or two in my thirties when I felt I had lost control of my emotions, I realized I was running from them in fear. Panic is probably a better word to describe what I was experiencing since I had associated those emotions with so much pain and shame. I felt out of control, and I couldn't seem to get a handle on myself, no matter how hard I tried. In reality, though, my emotions are just an alert system to let me know what's going on inside me. And just as I don't need to run from them, I also don't need to feed them. If they are not fed, they will die of starvation. Our thoughts are what feed and encourage our emotions. When we live in that place of feeding them, and then being ashamed of them, beating ourselves up for them, running away from them and denying that they exist, we create a never-ending cycle of defeat and discouragement.

I don't mean that we should be emotionless creatures. I believe we should embrace our emotions. But some emotions are harmful, especially when we chronically live in them. They don't lead us in the right direction. We hear a lot about trusting our gut. And today I'm a firm believer in trusting my intuition to make good decisions after I weigh the facts.

But learning how not to fight my emotions was huge for me. It gave me so much peace. I'm spending so much time talking about it here because we are often in the habit of hiding from our emotions without even realizing that's what we're doing. It becomes habitual behavior to do the things that help us cover them up. We do it subconsciously. That may mean reaching for the cookie jar when we are feeling stressed. It may mean zoning out in front of the TV with a bag of chips when we've had a rough day at work. I've seen so many examples of these coping mechanisms both in my life and the lives of the women I speak with. Sometimes, the initial phone call with me is the first time the woman on the other end of the line has taken a hard look at what she is really doing. She doesn't know why she is reaching for that bag of chips every night until we take a closer look at what's going on beneath the surface. Her coping mechanism is the bag of chips. It's how she is getting through life. And it's how she is managing, covering up, or running away from the negative emotions she's experiencing.

THE VIEW FROM INSIDE THE JAR

I've heard the same story dozens of times. We may be able to recognize these behaviors in others, but we can't see them in ourselves because we're too close to the situation and too much in our own heads. I love the saying "You can't read the label from inside the jar." We can't read the label of what we're doing, or thinking, because we're inside the jar. We can't get out of our own heads enough to see what's really going on. We look for solutions to the problems we're facing, which are more often than not only symptoms of the real problems. We think if only we could find that magic pill, the latest diet, or the newest gadget to tone our abs, we will be all right. We think the problem lies in the bag of chips, or the junk food our spouse brings into the house. We can google all day long, but we'll never see ourselves in all the advice we read because we're too close to our own situation. We're only looking at the back of the label, and it's blank. We can't step outside our own thought processes enough to see what's really going on.

That's why it's so easy to see what other people need to do, while not being able to grasp what we should be doing to set ourselves free. You might be thinking, "Oh, I know what I need to do, all right. I just don't do it." I've heard that one a hundred times, too. And that's exactly my point. We all have all the information we need to be fit and healthy and vibrantly happy. So, why aren't we? It's because we're stuck, and we don't know why we're stuck, or what might be holding us back. We're inside the jar.

My family and I recently added two new members to our household. I happened to see a post on Facebook about two parakeets who were in need of a new home. The owners had recently acquired a cat, and the cat was making a hobby of terrorizing the poor birds. They had been well loved and cared for up until the cat's arrival, and now it was evident to their family that they needed a new home.

As I write this, they've been in our home for a week. It's clear they've been traumatized, and it's easy to see why. Imagine being startled awake to see Shere Khan (from Rudyard Kipling's *The Jungle Book*) staring you in the face. The cat would suddenly spring up out of nowhere and grab onto the side of the cage with all four sets of claws. Apparently, this trauma had been going on, day and night, for a couple of months.

We don't have a way of telling our new friends that the cat isn't here and never will be here. They need to gradually learn a new story that it's safe to be in a darkened room, it's safe to sleep at night without having to be on high alert, and it's safe to be in other parts of their cage besides the topmost perch. It's okay to sing and play, and it's even okay to come out of their cage and fly around the room. Shere Khan is not coming back.

Puff and Rainbow have learned self-protective behaviors intended to keep them safe. But what they've really learned is how to be fearful and how to be unable to really live and enjoy their lives. They don't understand the danger has passed. In fact, their owners knew all along there was no real danger to them. They were in a cage, and the cat couldn't get in. But *they* don't know that they're okay. They're still living in danger mode. They definitely can't read the label, and they have no one who can tell them the truth. Only our careful nurturing of them, along with the healing effects of the passage of time, will bring them out of the prison of fear they're trapped in.

Bad things have happened to us. More than likely, bad things will happen to us in the future. But living constantly in that cage of fear makes those bad things the overarching theme of our life. We are reliving the past over and over again in our minds. We are projecting that past into a scary future for ourselves. We are constantly on high alert. We never know when we will open our eyes to see Shere Khan staring us in the face, sneering at us and licking his chops.

WE DON'T HAVE TO LIVE IN FEAR

But when we realize the fear we're experiencing is only a projection of what we believe will happen at some later point in time, we can understand we don't have to live there. We may feel as though there's no way out, but there is. We can do what Puff and Rainbow will never be able to do. We can question the stories we're telling ourselves and start living in a new reality. We don't have to see into the future to know that we're okay, right here and right now. We can know that everything that's happened in the past has brought us into this present moment. It all happened for us. We can live in this moment without reliving a traumatic past or projecting a terrifying future.

If we are present—present to our emotions and fears and the thoughts constantly flying through our heads—and we can learn stillness, we don't have to reach outside of ourselves to find peace. We don't have to flap wildly around our cage at the slightest trigger. We can know we are okay in this moment, and we will be okay in the next moment, too.

What's the thing you reach for to quiet those emotions of fear, shame, guilt, or whatever else they may be? Where do you retreat to when you're feeling tired, stressed, or discouraged? Now that you've identified the outward manifestation, and you're in that moment of truth—here I am doing this thing I know is destroying the life I want for myself—rather than giving in once again, just pause for a moment. Take a deep breath. What's really going on right now? What happened, and what old, worn-out thought pattern was triggered when that thing happened?

I encourage you in this moment just to be present to what's going on in your body. We feel our emotions in our body. They can cause us both physical pain and pleasure. It's that tightening of the throat. The knots in the stomach. The constriction in the chest that makes it hard to breathe. The elevated heart rate and blood pressure. No wonder we want to run from them! We don't have to be surprised that we want to cover them up and numb ourselves out to escape.

But I'm inviting you right now to take a moment to be present to them, instead of dashing out the nearest exit or flapping up to the highest perch in the cage. What are these physical feelings and the emotions that underlie them telling you? Start looking at them as windows into your subconscious mind. What happens when you are just still? When you're not quickly reaching for something outside yourself to shut them down? What if you began to experience them without shame and without fear?

EXPERIENCING PRESENCE

That's what I began to experience. Presence. And with that presence came a new freedom to forgive myself and love myself. And that is what ultimately opened the door to my freedom.

Allowing myself to be present with my emotions without shame, fear, or guilt allows me to begin to be free. There is a stillness of mind that comes with being present to my emotions. This allows me to be at peace in my own mind. And as I experience that peace, my clear mind can start to make better choices.

But we don't have to be quick to jump there, to the choices we can make once we are present to our emotions. First, let's take a look at what may be underlying those emotions. For every emotion we experience, at least one story can be attributed to it. What do I mean by a story? Let me start with the example of what has been identified as the biggest fear in our society today. Not death, not a devastating accident, not job loss or home foreclosure. What is it? The fear of public speaking. Yep. That's the number-one fear in our society today. If ever there was an emotion that came with a story, it's this one.

Let's take a look at it. Most of us have been talking since we were one or two years old. We didn't have to think too much about it; it just happened naturally. As we got older, we may have become more self-conscious about our speech, depending on how much we were corrected, or the level of support of our teachers and parents. But for most of us, no fear was associated with the act of speaking. We learned to fear it through some negative experience, usually of being ill-prepared and having to stand up in front of a room full of our peers. And then we got graded on how we did. Next time around, we procrastinated in our preparation a little bit more because that first experience registered in our subconscious as a negative one. We learned how to dread, and we put off thinking about it. That caused us to be even less prepared the second time around. Maybe we were so afraid of being judged or laughed at that we experienced actual physical illness, or maybe we manufactured that illness out of avoidance.

Our classifying of one task as "easy" and another as "hard" or even "terrifying" is all based on the stories we're telling ourselves. Our classmates' reaction when we gave our speech didn't have to fill us with embarrassment or shame. I'm not blaming us for taking it on, but that story never was about us. That was a story about those who were doing the ridiculing, just like if you ever ridiculed anyone, that was your story, not theirs. When I made some insulting comment to John, that only said something about me. It said nothing about John. If I hadn't heard myself say it, it would have just been a passing thought, and I would have forgotten all about it. That I still remember the incident (though I honestly don't remember the comment I made), tells me what a deep impression that experience had on me.

WHAT'S BEHIND YOUR STORY?

Here's why I keep referring to this phenomenon of the beliefs we hold onto about the past or the future as a story. A story is something we repeat. We derive some value from it. If we didn't, we wouldn't keep repeating it. Maybe we only repeat it to ourselves, playing it over and over again in our own mind. Maybe we repeat it to others. But we repeat it because it is important to us in some way. Maybe it allows us to be the victim. We get to indulge in self-pity when we repeat this story. It could be about a wrong done to us or circumstances that always seem to be against us. Maybe it's something we're proud of, and we replay it because it makes us feel good. Or maybe it's about something we did or neglected to do, to the detriment of someone else. Many of these stories fill us with shame and self-hatred. We may try to put them out of our minds, but they keep on floating back up to the surface.

Back to public speaking. The only difference between conversing comfortably with a close friend and standing on stage in front of a thousand people, besides the amount of preparation required, is the story we tell ourselves about these two situations. "All eyes are on me." So? There's a story behind that. The story is usually something along the lines of, *What if I trip while walking up to the podium? What if I faint? What if I forget my notes, or my mind goes blank, or my mouth is so dry that my tongue sticks to the roof of my mouth? What if I burp or suddenly get a bad case of the hiccups?* We feel as though we are under a microscope, and it fills us with terror. Just because I'm writing this doesn't mean I'm immune to it. Even as I type, with no public speaking events on the calendar, I can feel the butterflies waking up and starting to flutter in my stomach. Do you see the power of a story? You may never have to speak in front of an audience again in your life, yet when you read these words, you may have the same reaction I'm having right now.

But it's all just a story. We can think of anything as "hard" or "easy" based on the story we're telling ourselves. Our stories about public speaking just happen to be more vivid and deeply engrained than other stories we choose to tell ourselves. The thing is, we believe what we think. When we tell ourselves a story, our subconscious mind automatically starts to collect evidence for ways that story must be true. The more evidence we collect, the more inevitable the future outcome becomes to us. We have collected all the evidence to support the belief that "I'm horrible at public speaking." We may do all we can to avoid the possibility of having to speak in front of an audience, but in the event that we have to, we've got all the stories already in place to assure ourselves that we will fail miserably. And we've got all the fear and dread we need to be certain that not only will we be miserable during the event, but also for the entire time leading up to it, and most likely for a long time afterwards, too.

Those stories have their roots in the past, but then we carry them over into the dread of the future. Meanwhile, how much grief, ill health, squandered time, and additional weight have we put ourselves under, all because of some story that was anchored into our subconscious in the past, and that we have projected into our future? Think of how much stress Puff and Rainbow are under. We know there is no future threat. They are safe now. But their past history is causing them to live in fear of what may be waiting to pounce on them.

TURNING OUR STORIES AROUND

One of my coaches (and yes, I am fortunate enough to have several), Natasha, told me recently about how she was able to turn one of her stories around in such a way that it's had a huge positive effect on her entire household.

Natasha has a very busy work-from-home job (coaching being one of her responsibilities), besides being mom to four young kids. She would get to the end of a busy week and find that, once again, she hadn't managed to stay up on all the household chores. All those chores would be waiting for her on the weekend. She would be so disappointed in herself that she hadn't kept up on it, and she would tell herself the story at the end of each week that she had failed yet again. This disappointment would turn to anger that she couldn't get a handle on the chores.

Of course, this would put Natasha in a bad mood, and she would vent her anger on the tasks themselves in what her husband dubbed "rage cleaning." I know about rage cleaning—I can get a lot done if I clean when I am mad. But I don't recommend this method. Your peace and sanity are worth much more than getting your house cleaned a little more quickly.

Anyway, Natasha was in a routine of always being unhappy on the weekend due to feeling like a failure. Here's what finally turned this around: She decided that instead of viewing it as being behind, she would view it as preparing in advance for the week ahead. She would be going into the new week with everything sparkling and a feeling of being on top of things.

The kids now join in the cleaning extravaganza much more readily because they see they're contributing to something positive instead of picking up the pieces after a big failure. Natasha says it has completely changed her outlook on cleaning, and even her relationship with the rest of her family. Why be always feeling behind, when with a simple shift in thinking, she can be celebrating her beautiful clean home? Everyone is much happier with this shift. No more rage cleaning!

Going back to our public speaking example, what if instead of the old, worn-out stories that we've told ourselves over and over again, we came up with a new one? *Public speaking is my absolute favorite thing to do. Up on stage, speaking in front of a large audience, I love captivating them with my ideas and the flow of my words. I love the standing ovation I get at the end because I have so moved them. I love the emails, cards, and letters I get afterwards, thanking me and relating stories of how their lives have changed as a result of the speech I gave.* What if we imagine being elated with our accomplishment instead of going blank, stammering, and forgetting everything we wanted to say?

It changes everything when we approach our life—and it doesn't have to be anything as dreaded as public speaking—with joy, confidence, and enthusiasm. Anxiety and excitement are very closely related emotions. The only difference is how we frame an experience and how we view it. We can choose to be excited for the opportunity to stretch ourselves and grow, serve, and love. We don't have to cower in fear at life. We can allow ourselves to authentically be who we truly are on the inside.

"Okay, wait a minute, Lynn," you protest. "I am *not* a speaker. I am not going to get a standing ovation. Those cards and letters aren't coming in the mail. I can't tell myself lies. I can't live under such a delusion, only to be bitterly disappointed when all those delusions I've allowed myself to imagine don't come to fruition."

Okay, I get it. But let me ask you this: When was the last time the worst-case scenario you were expecting, that you built up so vividly in your mind, actually happened? I'll bet you didn't castigate yourself for lying to yourself. You may have been relieved, but you didn't say, "Wow, look at the delusion I was living under." You moved on with your life and came up with a new set of catastrophic beliefs about the next event on the horizon.

BEING STORY-FREE SETS US FREE

Isn't it time to be free? Wouldn't you love to be free? What if, instead of imagining ourselves falling flat on our face, and replaying that worst-case scenario over and over in our mind, we decided to tell ourselves a different story? I once read Susie Moore's book *What If It Does Work Out?* The title alone intrigued me. How many things do we hold ourselves back from for fear the circumstances won't work out in our favor? How many ideas have been crushed before they ever had a chance to see the light of day? Then we can ask ourselves, "What if I just flipped the story on its head? What if it all goes better than I could have imagined? What if it does work out? What would I do, who would I be, if I knew it was impossible to fail?"

Maybe you won't get a standing ovation. But what if in all your preparation, all the writing and revising and practicing, you were picturing those emails? What if you were picturing your audience lighting up with joy at your words? How would you show up differently to prepare? Maybe you would start to look forward to that prep time. Maybe you wouldn't procrastinate. It could change your entire approach and change the way you view the entire experience. And guess what? If you show up in dread and fear, and all your preparation has been eked out in dread and fear, your chances of inspiring your audience go down to almost zero.

Just to be clear, I'm not yet a public speaker. In fact, nobody is born a public speaker. It's a skill that can be learned just like everything else. This is not a book about public speaking. (You may have been starting to wonder.) I'm using public speaking as an illustration to help you see that when you approach your life, your health, your household tasks, or whatever, with a defeatist attitude, you are almost guaranteed to keep right on going on that exact same unpleasant path you've been on. Yet one simple shift in thinking can change everything. And I mean everything.

Changing your life can be as simple as changing the story you're telling yourself.

QUESTIONS FOR REFLECTION

What characteristics or identity do you want to live in?
_____
_____
_____
_____

What do you no longer wish to be defined by?
_____
_____
_____
_____

Do you use a coping mechanism to deal with your emotions, or are you able to be still and experience them?
_____
_____
_____
_____

What stories are you telling yourself when it comes to something you fear? What is your Shere Khan?
_____
_____
_____
_____

Chapter 6

Turning Our Stories Upside Down

In the last chapter, I described how caught up in stories we can become without even realizing it. It can be quite eye-opening to understand we constantly tell ourselves stories. We are story-making machines. We have a story for everything. I've been working on my stories for a few years now, and I'm still finding them running through my mind all the time.

The difference is that now I'm not ruled by them. Once you learn to recognize your stories, and you have started to live in a different place than the land of endless stories, you will be on that path to freedom, too. It can help to start with the biggest and most prevalent story in your life. If you start with the one most in the forefront of your mind, subsequent stories that come up start to get easier to deal with.

I had known for some time, even several years after my divorce, that my ex-husband was taking up way too much real estate in my head. I didn't want to keep being controlled by him. The truth is, I wasn't being controlled by him at all. I was being controlled by my choice to continually relive incidents from the past.

Here I was, in my late fifties, with a beautiful, happy, peaceful life I was so grateful for, living in the past. My mind was not at peace, despite all I had done to rebuild my life.

Earlier, I told you I had been a mom and wife, raising and homeschooling our six children in the mountains of Idaho. Our house was perched on top of a steep hill, and out our windows, we had a panoramic vista of the surrounding mountains. When I stepped out my front door, I was in nature. It was the closest thing we could get to wilderness, while still enjoying the benefits of civilization.

My husband built our house himself, from the ground up, on a very low budget. Really, what we were building was a dream. It was an ideal we were living into of being able to raise our children the way we wanted and to allow them the freedom to learn and explore. I thoroughly enjoyed homeschooling them, and I am so grateful I had that opportunity.

I realized, though, somewhere in the midst of homeschooling, that the dream was beginning to crumble around me. My idyllic life was dying before my very eyes, and it was all I could do to try to hold it together each day. What was my dream? Being able to look back after having raised our six kids into adulthood with an intact marriage and family. Having our adult children bring our grandchildren to their childhood home to play and roam in the hills as they had done growing up. That was the image I held in my mind. To have my children be the product of just another failed marriage and broken family was the last thing I wanted for them. And the last thing I wanted for myself.

After having held that dream so closely to my heart for so many years, a major incongruence occurred in my subconscious thoughts when I found myself living a completely different life in my fifties. My brain and my heart were still trying to make sense of it all. I realized somewhere along the line that this endless replaying of stories was my subconscious mind's way of seeking to piece it all together. How did this happen? How did I get here? I somehow thought if I replayed it all enough times, I would finally understand, make sense of it all, and find peace.

I knew I wasn't seeking validation from others because I rarely talked about these things. My need to rehash it all to others had died down a few years prior. My ex, after I left home, considered it his duty to make sure everyone understood his side of the story so his reputation would remain intact. He would let me know, "*Everyone* agrees with me." So be it. I was okay with that. But what I was seeking in rehashing my stories over and over again to myself was the validation to my inner self. I was internally trying to fit it all together. Why was I here, leading such a different life, one so foreign to the path I had been on for so many years? I thought I would live in that amazing place for the rest of my life. I even joked that I wanted to be buried there on my little piece of heaven on earth. Everything in my new life was a far cry from what I had planned.

Those replays of the old scenes—and there were a lot of them—became the summer reruns of my mind. Words that had been spoken to me, ways that I had been treated. How I had been silenced and devalued. The constant replay became like the emotional addiction I had experienced so many years prior. The more I tried to get the unpleasantness out of my mind, the more forefront it became. I might do all right for a while, but then some phrase, some minor, completely innocent action of a random person would remind me of a way I had been treated, some injustice I had endured, and off I would go, replaying the whole scene in my mind once again.

Even though my days of feeling powerless were behind me, I still was not in control of my own thoughts. I had a brand new life. I was happy; I had a kind and caring husband, a secure financial situation, and a stable job as an RN, but I was still trapped in my own head.

When I could finally let go of my need to constantly prove to myself that I had done the right thing, when I could truly forgive and put it all in the past, I knew I was free. As I had experienced earlier in my life, after having been in prison, freedom feels really good. I didn't try to forget it all. Yes, I can still remember incidents from the past. I can still remember unkind words that were spoken to me. I didn't suddenly develop amnesia. For better or worse, I've got a great memory. The difference now is I no longer have the need to rehearse and rehash. I have nothing to prove to myself. I now know nothing happens to me; it only happens for me. It took a lot for me to leave my dream home, in my dream location, and the marriage I had invested so many years of my life into. But every single thing I have experienced happened *for* me. Each little thing, and each big thing, brought me to this beautiful place in which I find myself now. It took drastic measures to dislodge me from my former dream. I went kicking and screaming, figuratively speaking.

Now I'm just grateful. I love my life. And I wouldn't be here today if not for all the difficulties I went through. When the thoughts pop back into my head that used to take me to a chaotic state and keep me there, instead of fighting them or ignoring or stuffing them, I'm grateful. All I can say is "Thank you. It doesn't matter what your intent was. I forgive you. I forgive myself. You helped to make me into who I am today. You have given me the resolve to succeed and be my very best self. You've put a message in my heart that I can share with the world. It is an incredible gift that you've given me. And again I thank you. I embrace what is."

And I don't mean that in a sarcastic or vengeful kind of way. I sincerely mean it. When we're really free and we're loving our life, how can we regret anything from our past? It all brought us here, to this beautiful present.

"But, Lynn," you might protest, "my present is far from beautiful. I'm up to my ears in difficulties and stress. I have no idea how I'm going to make it financially."

AM I OKAY RIGHT NOW?

And here is what I've learned to ask myself, when those kinds of stories come up: *What do I need right now, just to exist in this moment? What do I need that I don't already have? Am I okay right now? Do I need anything just to sit here and breathe?*

When I ask myself that calmly and honestly, a peace floods my body in even the most stressful of situations. My mind clears. And I can then make a plan and choose the next right action.

I first really experienced this peace a couple of years ago. Through the reading (and by reading, I primarily mean listening to audio books, at least for the last two years or so) I had been doing to start my business, Be Fit Beyond Fifty, I was introduced to the work of Byron Katie. I had never heard of her before, but I was intrigued by what another author had to say about her after he had met her personally. He had been deeply impacted by her teaching. I immediately found an audio book by her and started listening.

As of this writing, I have probably listened at least ten times to her book *Your Inner Awakening* (available only on Audible). I instantly fell in love with it because it meshed so well with what I had already found in my own life, and what I was teaching my clients. What I learned from Byron Katie was how to simplify and streamline the process of becoming at peace with oneself, along with how to go deep with it. She gives a simple process for turning any story around and giving yourself the gift of a peaceful, joyful life. I have woven her practice into my own life and teaching, and I am deeply grateful to her for what it has meant to myself and others.

One evening a couple of years ago, I was driving home by myself from Boise, the city nearest to us, to Cascade, the small town of 900 where we live. It's about a ninety-minute drive on a beautiful, winding mountain highway. We had purchased my husband's truck a few months prior, but I was unfamiliar with it since I had not yet driven it much. Driving along, listening to Byron Katie and enjoying the breathtaking scenery, I noticed a flash of red on the dash. By the time I glanced down, the light was off again. This happened several times before I focused on it. *Oh, no. It's the check oil light.* The dealer had told us the truck had been serviced and was ready to go, and we hadn't put many miles on it since then. I was completely unprepared. The road being what it was, it took me a while to reach a turnout where I could pull safely off the highway. I parked next to the river in the steep canyon. I have a AAA membership, but it doesn't do me much good when there is no cell service. I felt the panic rise up within me. I was still many miles from home, and I didn't want to blow up the engine on Ross's new truck. There weren't many cars going past on a weekday evening. I had no spare quarts of oil in the truck.

What was I going to do? The words of Byron Katie I had just been listening to went through my head. She had been talking about one particularly pervasive story that we tell ourselves: *I need money.* I knew I didn't need money right in that moment. What I thought I needed was oil for our truck. But as I sat there contemplating my situation, I realized I didn't need anything. I was safely parked. I had food because I had just done the grocery shopping while in town. I even had some bedsheets from my father-in-law's house that I was bringing back to our house. I had everything I needed to sit there, right in that moment, and I had so much more than I needed. I relaxed. And from that place of stillness and gratitude, I made a plan.

Maybe it wasn't the best plan, but it didn't have to be. It was much better than any plan I could have made in a state of panic. I found a piece of paper and a pen, and I wrote out my information and the AAA number. I would flag down a car and ask the driver to make a call for me when they got in range of cell coverage. AAA would come, maybe an hour or two or three later, and get me out of my predicament. They aren't known for being fast in my neck of the woods, but they do come through.

I waited for a car to come around the bend, and I waved my arms in the air. They drove past without glancing in my direction. No worries.

After several minutes, another vehicle rounded the bend, and I waved my arms again. This one pulled over. It was an older man with his adult daughter. I explained my predicament. He had oil with him. I hadn't actually checked the oil level yet; I had just trusted what the idiot light was telling me. The stick was dry. I tried to turn the cap, but it was stuck. I couldn't budge it. Even the strong mountain man couldn't budge it. He rummaged in his truck and found a crowbar and a hammer. He placed the crowbar on the finger ridges of the cap and pounded it with the hammer.

It took a while, but it finally loosened up enough to come unscrewed. He kindly filled the tank with two quarts of oil. He noticed that my coolant tank was pretty much empty also. Yes, he had coolant, too. He emptied it into the reservoir. I searched in my wallet for cash to give him, and only came up with $13. He took it with a shrug. I wish I had thought to write him a check, or maybe even give him some groceries, because I knew he gave me more than $13 worth of oil and coolant. I started up the truck and it sounded fine. They were going farther than the turnoff to my house, but they told me to follow them until I turned off the highway to make sure the truck was okay. I thanked them profusely and followed them up the highway, waving as I turned off to my road. I was grateful beyond words.

CHOOSING CALM

That day I realized something. I could have approached that situation in two different ways: fear and panic, or calm and presence. Would the outcome have changed if I had been terrified? Maybe not. Maybe if my hands were shaking and my heart was pounding, it would make for a more interesting story now. Maybe I would have thought that without cell service, I had no choice but to drive the rest of the way home and risk destroying the engine. Who knows what I would have thought? I do know I would have been mentally and emotionally exhausted when I finally made it home. Instead, I felt as if I had taken a pleasant drive through the country, with a peaceful stop along the Payette River, which in actuality is what I did. And I got my truck filled up with oil along the way, due to the kindness of strangers. As a side note, today I check that truck before we drive it, and I make sure we've got a spare quart or two of oil stashed behind the driver's seat. You never know when that might come in handy, and it never hurts to be prepared.

And here's the biggest takeaway. In that story, nothing bad or even slightly uncomfortable ever happened. If I had given way to panic, my default response, it would have been completely based on my imaginings of a scary future. It would have been a story I was telling myself of something I feared would happen. We have a tendency to automatically catastrophize our future. We believe the story we're telling ourselves, and it fills us with fear and terror about something that is not happening, and probably never will.

Does that mean that if we are present in the moment, nothing bad will ever happen to us? Obviously, bad things still happen. But no matter what is happening, how much pain we're in, or what kind of devastating circumstance we find ourselves in, if we can look within and be honest with ourselves, the answer to the question, "Am I okay right in this moment?" will be yes. Maybe it will only be yes 99 percent of the time. I will grant you that. But so much of our suffering is caused by what we think is going to happen, not by what is actually happening right now. And if we know that, we can drastically reduce the suffering we experience.

OUR THOUGHTS FEED OUR EMOTIONS

But what if we are living in a constant flood of negative emotions and feel like there is no escape? My emotional addiction was caused by the thoughts I chose. My thoughts continued to feed it, and then it became an endless cycle. For me, the emotions themselves were the addiction. And the thoughts and emotions were based on the story I was telling myself.

Some of my clients have a really hard time with this. What if the story is true? I can't change reality and stop believing something that really happened to me. And if it really happened, how can I call it a story?

It's true we can't change things that factually happened in time and space. We may wish we could rewind the clock and go back and change history, but we know that's impossible. And we don't want to just stuff the memories and try to put them out of our minds. But we can change the frame we put around the story. That's what I did when I realized everything that's happened to me wasn't really *to* me. It was *for* me. My frame up until a few years ago was my victim status. When I was in my first marriage, I made it my practice to fly under the radar as much as I possibly could. I did my best to avoid unpleasant situations. But those unpleasant situations kept happening. That was the reality. Yet I was the one who took those incidents personally and put my own interpretation on them. I created a story around them.

As I said earlier, it was never about me. But even though it wasn't about me, it was *for* me. I don't blame myself for not understanding that at the time. I don't blame myself for taking on the victim mentality or for feeling powerless to change the situation. I acted according to what I believed. Now I have a new frame to put around every single incident I remember from my past. And that frame is gratitude. When I look back on a story with gratitude, it changes the story. When I know any particular incident brought me to this place in my life and made me who I am now, there is no room for regret, bitterness, or unforgiveness. There is no room for shame.

ARE WE FOOLING OURSELVES?

I'd better ask this question again to make sure I'm as clear as I can be. How can I believe something that's not true? I can't pretend something is true when I know it's not. But there is a positive and a negative side to everything. We don't have to believe the negative any more than we have to believe the positive. The positive belief is there for the taking, no matter how dire our current situation may look. Both beliefs are available to us at any given time.

As an example, let's take working out. We can see our waistline growing, and we can see our cardiovascular health diminishing. We can see it used to be easy to walk up the stairs, and now we are gasping for air. So we know we should exercise, but that thought fills us with dread because we have held onto the idea that we hate exercise. Our thoughts may run like this: "Exercise is hard. It hurts. I don't have enough energy. I don't have enough time. I don't have the right equipment or the space or the know-how to have a proper workout. I will do it wrong. If I work out today, I know I will be blowing it off in a week, if not by tomorrow. So why even start? If anyone finds out I'm even thinking about exercise, they will laugh because I have failed so many times already. Then I will feel even more shame than I did before I started. I will embarrass myself. And that will discourage me even more." Perhaps, like my sister Terri, you have exercise-induced asthma. Exercising is associated with being unable to breathe, which triggers all your survival mechanisms. It becomes not just unpleasant, but traumatic to set off that response in your body.

You didn't know you had so many negative beliefs about exercise, did you? No wonder you procrastinate. Maybe you were picked last for the kickball team in elementary school. It really doesn't matter where this story came from. This is not therapy. All we need to do is recognize that yes, this is a story we are telling ourselves. We can recognize that this story is no longer serving us, that we are so much better off without this story. Then we can learn how to turn it around.

How do we turn it around? We boil our story down to a simple statement, and we start playing with it in our mind by turning it upside down from its original meaning.

We look for even just one example of how the opposite statement is as true or truer than the original. As Byron Katie says, if you can find one example, you can find two. Then, if you can find two, you can find three. When you've found three examples, your mind is opened up to a new world of possibilities. This is how we free ourselves from all the old thinking patterns that have been keeping us stuck.

The original statement was "I hate to exercise." Now we take the opposite. We tend to think of the opposite of hate as love, but we don't need to take it that far if that causes a pushback on the inside. The simplest and most direct opposite would be, "I *don't* hate to exercise." That's a start! When I'm working with my clients, I always start with helping the person I'm speaking with to perhaps redefine exercise. Maybe the concept of exercise could be expanded to include gardening or dancing. Just maybe you can remember a time when walking in your neighborhood led to a fun reconnecting with a neighbor you hadn't seen in a year. Maybe there was a time when you went on a hike and the scenery was so gorgeous and you felt so invigorated that you forgot to call it exercise.

Remember, we only need three real examples of times when you loved to exercise or at least tolerated it reasonably well. Do you have your three? Great! Now when your mind goes back to that idea, *I hate to exercise*, there will be a little jolt in your subconscious mind. *Wait a minute; I can remember times when that was not true.* As you allow those new beliefs to simmer in your subconscious mind, you will find new attitudes forming. Maybe instead of being so quick to dismiss the idea of exercise, you will start to act on the new beliefs.

My sister Terri quite understandably had a strong aversion to feeling unable to breathe. She associated being sedentary in the comfortable, climate-controlled environment of her home with safety. Movement such as going for a walk would bring on the wheezing, and with it came the fear. There are people out walking their dogs, and she is severely allergic to animal dander. More fear. Her story became, "I don't go outside. I don't do things. I stay home." Her story went so far as, "Everyone else has a life. I don't have a life. I won't be interesting to all these people who are out living their lives. I won't have anything to talk about with them, and I will bore them."

Together, we have turned these stories around. Since becoming my client, Terri has lost a significant amount of weight and kept it off (another story defeated!) and moderate exercise is no longer bringing on the asthma. Besides learning that she could take a deep breath without hurting herself or setting off the asthma response, she has been able to build her stamina and endurance. She has redefined her identity as "someone who goes outside and does things." She loves her new life, and her husband is thrilled that she now wants to go on walks, travel, and explore. "Oh, you go ahead, and I'll see you when you get home," has turned into, "Yes, let's go!" She's on a new path, all because she started telling herself new stories. The old stories don't make any sense anymore. A tiny shift in thinking led to a monumental result.

BREAKING FREE

Byron Katie has written entire books on the subject of breaking free of the stories we're telling ourselves. However, as much as I've recommended her books to people, very few have really grabbed onto this idea of being free in our own minds and experienced the full benefit of this teaching. Instead, they stay stuck in their old stories. That's why I love having this teaching as part of the transformation process I bring to my coaching clients. They get to experience the beauty of this process as it applies to their particular circumstance and their stories, with someone who really understands what's going on under the surface. Sometimes the realizations happen in an instant, and I get the joy of seeing a huge breakthrough in my client. Other times, it comes in many slow understandings over a longer period of time. Either way, the transformation is a beautiful thing to behold.

Personally, I have learned that just about all my passing thoughts boil down to a story I am telling myself. It's either a story about the past or a story about the future. The stories about the past are what fuel our shame, guilt, regret, anger, and bitterness. Of course, we can have happy memories about the past, too, and I heartily encourage those. But those are not usually the stories keeping us stuck and driving us into binge eating, emotional attachments, and other dependencies.

Our stories about the future can fill us with dread, anxiety, fear, and even terror. When a client comes to me with that kind of a story, I gently remind her that this terrifying future hasn't happened yet. It only exists in her mind. And she will often say, "Yes, but I know it's going to happen." That is when I gently encourage her to open up some new possibilities for herself. We have a tendency to take the worst-case scenario and blow it up in our minds to the point of panic. The thing we are focused on is the thing most likely to happen. So let's focus on the positive and watch beauty begin to unfold in our lives.

LEARNING TO VISUALIZE

I talk a lot about envisioning a bright, amazing future for yourself. Many of my clients have a hard time visualizing. What I have realized and what I tell them now is they really don't have a hard time visualizing. If you have ever been so gripped with fear of all the bad things that could happen to you in a particular scenario that your heart starts racing and your mouth goes dry, then you have not only visualized it, but you have also emotionalized it. It is so real in your own mind that you can't imagine it not taking place.

Now, we want to take that scary future and turn it from worst-case scenario to best-case scenario. What would be the very best thing that could happen in this instance? Remember, the picture we are holding in our minds is the one more likely to happen. Why is that? Because we act according to what we tell ourselves. If we are acting out of fear and panic, we are not making the best choices we possibly could for ourselves. We are living out our very own self-fulfilling prophecy. What? You didn't know you were a prophet? When we live in worry, we are creating the conditions for the things we are worried about to occur, at least when those occurrences are the result of our own actions, or lack of action.

LEAVING PERFECTIONISM BEHIND

I'm a big advocate of us all living our best lives. Let's embrace life in all its messiness, instead of being so afraid of messing it up. We can start living our best life today. The problem comes when we start thinking that living our best life means we have to be perfect. We are never going to be perfect. We are imperfect beings. We can understand that intellectually, but it can still be a blind spot for us. It's easy to let our need to be perfect keep us stuck in imperfection. We tell ourselves, *I know I can't be perfect, so why even bother? I intended to stay away from the cookies today, and instead, I ate the whole box. Since I've already blown it for today, I'll go ahead and eat this donut that's been calling my name, too. I'll start over again tomorrow.* Tomorrow comes and all the same patterns play out on repeat. And then we throw up our hands in despair and give up. *See, you knew you couldn't do it. Why did you even try?* And thus begins again that continuous cycle of attempting huge changes all at once, failing, giving up, and falling back into despair.

That's how perfectionism keeps us stuck. I see it over and over again in myself and in my clients. It's easy to set goals that are too big and lofty for our current state of mind and our current mental or physical muscle. When we set a goal that's too big, it leads to procrastination. Our subconscious mind wants to keep us safe. When it senses that hesitation, that little bit of fear that rises up when we are about to start something new, the alarms go off in our subconscious mind and we think of all kinds of reasons we should be doing something else right now.

So we turn back to the comfortable and the familiar. We procrastinate. We don't understand why we are procrastinating. And then we start to think it's because we really don't care. We must not really want it badly enough. If we had more willpower or motivation, surely we would succeed. We must not have what it takes. We become so afraid of failure because we perceive that we have failed so many times in the past. And every time we start up again, our minds only throw up more evidence for why we can't succeed, and why we will never succeed. We start to believe that story, and we stay stuck.

How can we set ourselves free from perfectionism? First of all, know that you are not alone. Even just admitting that we have perfectionistic tendencies inside us is a key step to freedom. Many of us who have fallen prey to addictions are perfectionistic by nature. And then we, as perfectionists, tend to become really great procrastinators. Rather than labeling myself as a procrastinator, which I refuse to do any more, by the way, I now view it as a problem in implementation.

I envision the beautiful life I want for myself. I am filled with gratitude for the beautiful life I already have. I outline the long-term goals I need to set my sights on to accomplish my vision. I don't try to change everything all at once. I take those long-term goals and break them down into smaller weekly and then daily goals. I keep my daily goals very small and realistic. I surround myself with the support and accountability I need to keep me on the path. And then I look very carefully at that daily goal. It may still be too big. It's the consistent effort, day in and day out, that wins the race. It's not a sprint. We won't get to the finish line all at once.

BREAKING IT DOWN

One of my favorite mantras as I was training for my first marathon was "You can't cram for a marathon." My former habit of leaving a major term paper for the last two days of the semester and then working like crazy on it just doesn't work when training for a marathon. That's where I learned that just a little bit of consistency each day pays big dividends.

Even our daily goals can be broken down into tiny steps. Make each step so tiny that you feel no resistance to it at all. Instead of, *I will walk two miles*, your tiny step can be, *I will put on my shoes*. There is nothing for your subconscious mind to freak out about over putting on your shoes. There's no need to think about the whole two miles or two blocks or whatever the distance is. Once the shoes are on, you can simply tell yourself you're just going to put on your jacket, if needed, and step outside.

Ahh, once you're outside, take a deep breath. Don't start arguing with yourself that you're not dressed properly or that you're too tired or any other excuse. Just put one foot in front of the other. And you're walking! That wasn't so bad, was it? Don't allow yourself to think, *Oh, I have to do this every day*. Don't start thinking, *This is so hard. I have so many other things I should be doing.* Remember that this activity is one tiny step closer to the life you are envisioning for yourself. Smile!

All of our goals can be approached in this way. We are not eating the whole elephant all at once. One step at a time, one bite at a time. Tell yourself you no longer have a need to procrastinate. You can go so far as to thank procrastination for how it has served you, and then say goodbye. The same with perfectionism. You no longer have to be perfect. When you do something or you don't do something and you perceive it as failure, don't beat yourself up. It just means you're human. Pick yourself up and get right back on the wagon. If you need to adjust or readjust your tiny steps or goals, go right ahead. There is no right or wrong here. There is joy in this journey. There is joy in learning how to be kind to yourself. There is joy in giving yourself the very best self-care you possibly can.

How would it feel to be free of the stories you are telling yourself? No matter how little imagination or creativity you think you have, you are always telling yourself stories. And so am I. We can never truly be story free because we are story-making machines. We can't help ourselves. But what we can help is what type of story we tell ourselves. Stay tuned, because that's what we'll be exploring next.

QUESTIONS FOR REFLECTION

How can you put a new frame around the stories you tell yourself?
_____
_____
_____
_____

What do you procrastinate on? What stories do you tell yourself about those tasks you put off?
_____
_____
_____
_____

How can you start telling yourself a new story about that task?
_____
_____
_____
_____

Give three examples of how the new belief is as true or truer than the original story.
_____
_____
_____
_____

Chapter 7

Valuing Ourselves Means Living in Joy

I had never heard of Sean Stephenson before I had the privilege of hearing him speak at a live event. He had the most striking appearance of anyone I have ever met. I believe that is partially because very few people with his condition, osteogenesis imperfecta, live past very early childhood, at least in such severe cases as his. In fact, the doctors attending to him at birth told his parents they should start preparing for his death because chances were very slim that he would make it past the first 24-48 hours of life.

As a result of his disease, Sean experienced stunted growth and used a wheelchair for mobility. In his talk that day, he jokingly compared himself to a bug, with a small, oval-shaped body with tiny arms and legs, and a normal-sized head. If he could have stood, he would have been three feet tall. But his fragile legs could not support the weight of his body. Instead, as he delivered the most inspirational talk I've ever heard, he strode confidently back and forth across the stage, using his arms to propel his manual wheelchair.

Everyone in the audience was mesmerized by Sean. He exuded the most confidence I have ever witnessed. He had us rocking with laughter. He never once asked or even hinted that we pity him. He loved life and reached for his dreams as boldly as anyone possibly could. He was one of the conference's final speakers, and he left an indelible impression on my mind. He left us all as he wanted to leave us, with the understanding that if he could overcome insecurity and self-doubt and learn to face the disbelief and stares of others with humor and grace, we could do the same.

I heard Sean speak in March 2018. I fully intended to attend one of his speaking workshops that August, but unfortunately, it didn't work out for me. Now I deeply regret not making the extra effort it would have taken to get there. He passed away a year later at the age of forty, dying as a result of head injuries caused by a fall. His last words were to his wife, Mindy: "This didn't happen to me; it happened for me."

That philosophy summed up how Sean lived his life, and how he finally faced death. He was an inspiration to me because despite the tremendous obstacles he faced, he saw the good in life and chose to live it to his fullest capacity. Besides being a motivational speaker since his late teens, he earned a degree in political science and even went on to obtain a doctoral degree in clinical hypnotherapy. He had his own therapy practice, driven by the need to provide guidance to those who came to him seeking help for their own insecurities. He was known as the three-foot giant, and that title suited him well.

Sean was such an inspiration to me because I am well acquainted with the prison of insecurity and the feeling that I'm "not enough." If Sean could live a full and courageous life, why can't I? And truly, that was the heart of his message.

Nothing happens to us; it only happens for us. When we really begin to believe this, it changes everything. It takes us out of "why me?" mode and puts us into gratitude. How does it do that? Adopting this belief that everything happens for our ultimate good puts us into a different frame of mind. It puts us in the attitude of looking for the lesson in every circumstance. When we carry this attitude around with us, it puts us on the lookout for what we can learn from this situation. We start looking for that silver lining in the dark cloud.

If Sean had been born without that severe birth defect, would I have ever heard of him? Would he have risen above the average challenges all of us face and brought himself to the level of being able to inspire millions? My guess is he would have lived an average life, with an average job, earning an average living. It's the resistance he faced, and his attitude toward it, that made him great.

All we really need to do when we are facing a difficult situation is to ask ourselves, "Do I have what I need to live right now in this moment?" If we ask ourselves that question honestly, the answer will always be yes. Even in the most chaotic of moments, we can find stillness and peace within ourselves. Doing so may seem impossible, but when we put it into practice in the here and now, in the current moment we are living in, we find that "yes" within ourselves.

OPENING THE DOOR TO GRATITUDE

When we are living into a scary future that hasn't happened yet is when we find ourselves lacking. If we are living in the current moment, we will find we are okay. And this opens the door for gratitude. I am a spiritual person, and I find my faith resting in God. But spiritual beliefs aside, you can look within and find this to be true. You have what you need, right now, to live in this moment, and the next one, and the one after that. If you take the time to be present, there will never come a moment when you do not find this to be true.

Even if you have no one or nothing to express gratitude to, the mere act of being grateful opens up new pathways in your brain. It releases the feel-good chemicals into your bloodstream. You start to experience life with a whole new outlook. And you find yourself replacing chaos with peace.

You start learning how to view life through the eyes of abundance rather than scarcity. You start to realize everything is going to be okay. You discover that it was your hyper-focus on the worry and fear of something that hasn't happened yet that caused all your unhappiness. When a new situation arises, you begin to face it with resourcefulness.

This doesn't only help with worries about the future. It also opens up the door to approaching our past with gratitude. As I told you earlier, only a few years ago, I was plagued with stories about my past. I would remember wrongs that had been done to me, and I would replay them over and over again in my mind. I would try to clear my mind of them, and then some new incident or something someone said would trigger a memory, and there I was back again in the old stories.

What finally turned this situation around for me was learning how to live in abundance and embrace the present moment. When I realized nothing happens to me and it all happens for me, and when I experienced true forgiveness for myself and others at a deep level, I was able to approach my past with gratitude. If I really, truly believe everything happens for my ultimate good, then how can I approach those memories with anger or resentment? How can I spend even a single moment in regret when everything in the past has brought me to the beautiful, abundant life I'm living right now?

When we live in gratitude for our past, our story about that past changes. We realize the story we were hanging onto, in which we were the helpless victim, actually is not true. As our beliefs begin to align with this new reality, we begin to be changed from the inside out. Now, in my mind, whenever one of those old memories floats to the surface, I say thank you to the person who spoke the words or did the actions I had mistakenly thought were against me. What I realize is that whatever anybody did, that action was based on a story they were telling themselves. That other person is full of stories just like I was. They were acting out of their own faulty belief system, what they believed to be true. They believed what they thought, and that caused them to act in the way they did. It was never about me. Any act perpetrated against us is not about us at all. It's all a story the other person is believing.

NO LONGER THE VICTIM

When I understand it's not about me, I am no longer the victim. I am the bystander to the story that someone else is believing. I don't have to take that story on myself and receive it as something that is true about me. When it's not about me, forgiveness becomes a much simpler task. I can forgive myself that I was only believing my thoughts. I believed my thoughts to be true, and I believed the story that emerged out of those thoughts to be true. When I understand this, I experience self-forgiveness. And then I find that the other person's stories are really not so different from my own. So I can forgive them for believing their stories also.

This is incredibly freeing when you allow it to be so. We don't have to be caught in the trap of reliving all the wrongs that have been done to us or by us. We can be free. Now when I spiral down into victimhood once again, I only need to remember how that thing I thought was a wrong against me brought me to where I am now and molded me into the person I am now. I remember that everything happens for me. And I am grateful.

As I write this, I can hear the protests. "Lynn, you haven't experienced what I went through. The magnitude of what I have endured is so much greater than anything you have faced in your life. You can't begin to imagine it." I can affirm that is probably true. But the thing is we each have our own path to travel. We can allow evil to triumph by retreating into victimhood, or we can rise up victorious out of the wreckage. The choice is open to us either way, and it is ours for the taking in any given moment. Victim and victor are both available for the taking anytime we want them. Which would you rather live in? Wouldn't you rather know that everything, no matter how tragic or devastating that thing is, has molded you into who you are at this moment and brought you to this beautiful life that lies open before you right now?

If anyone had an excuse to retreat into victimhood, it was Sean Stephenson. He looked *different* in every sense of the word. I am so grateful he had parents who didn't hold him back in any way but allowed him to soar and be his absolute best. I know that took a lot of courage on their part. It would have been so much easier to surround him with pillows and do everything in their power to keep him safe. Next time you are tempted to lapse into self-consciousness or shame over your appearance, your intelligence, or any ability you feel yourself lacking in, I invite you to look up Sean at YouTube and be inspired by one of his videos. Sean used what he had been given to achieve the unimaginable. He mastered insecurity and self-doubt to the point that they were non-existent in his life. If he could do it, so can you.

As for me, now I get to live in joy and abundance. My "not enoughness" has disappeared. That doesn't mean I don't slip back into my old ways. It doesn't mean I don't get angry or frustrated or irritated. It does mean I get to see the choice laid out before me in each moment. Because I now live most of my waking moments in abundance, gratitude, and joy, the frustration, anger, worry, and any other negative emotions that come up are no longer congruent with where I am living. And I see in that moment that once again I have that choice. I can hang onto those negative emotions, or I can let them go. I'd much rather let them go. When I hang onto them, I'm the one who suffers. It's really not about anyone else, any more than their story is about me.

FINDING A WAY

I have told you how I have shifted my thinking about my past. One thing I'm very grateful for is my resourcefulness. Because we never had much money as we were raising our children, I learned to be very frugal. This mindset came easily for me because I was raised by my dad to be frugal. But my dad's frugality came from his upbringing. Ours, in my early adult life, was out of necessity. I learned how to be very resourceful, especially in the area of cooking. I knew we didn't have much money, often no money, but there was always food to put on the table. Even though we had very little money, I never thought of us as poor.

I'm not sure why, or where this came from, but no matter how little money I had, I loved investing in self-development. We found a way to make music lessons happen for the kids and scraped together the money for 4-H and other activities. It's a very normal thing for parents to sacrifice for their kids' education and enrichment. The thing that seems a bit different is I had some sort of deeply ingrained need to make sure I continued learning and developing even as an adult. It would not have been super-unusual, I realize now, for me to have just told myself we didn't have the money for anything for me and left it at that. But I pushed through and found a way to make it happen.

Looking back, I am so grateful for all the pushback I received. Now I know that was one of the best things that could have happened to me. Would I have ever come up with the same level of determination and persistence if not for my husband's pushback? I really don't think so.

The resistance kept me out of apathy. My husband never forbade me to run, but he did put quite a bit of effort into guilt manipulation to try to dissuade me from running. The same with my attempts to start a business or to better myself in some way. Looking back, I'm so grateful for that resistance. I learned in running up big hills that resistance was a good thing, but I never realized until recently how much the resistance I faced in my marriage also made me stronger.

I know I wouldn't have achieved the level I did in my running without the physical hills I faced every day. But even more so, the psychological barriers of having someone who considered himself "above" me, telling me I "shouldn't" run, or I shouldn't be better than him in anything, because that was disrespectful and would cause me to be prideful, only served to fuel my resolve to do what was in my heart to do. I didn't care about being better or faster than anyone else. I was doing it for me.

Throughout college, I noticed I tended to get higher grades in the classes I thought would be more difficult for me. The ones I thought would be easy were the ones I would slack off in. In the same way, if I thought I had all kinds of time, I would distract myself and not get much done. If I was under a time crunch, usually due to my chronic procrastination, I would suddenly become ultra-efficient and productive, and power through mammoth amounts of work in a short amount of time.

The lesson here is we need resistance to thrive. Whenever the task that lay before me was hard, I would rise to the challenge. When I thought it was going to be easy, I would become apathetic and not do nearly as well. These days, whatever form the resistance takes, I'm learning to embrace it with gratitude.

NOBODY CARES

Another surprising, but freeing, thing I learned during that time was the idea that *nobody cares*. On the surface, that sounds self-pitying, as in, "I think I'll go out to the backyard and eat some worms." But no, I mean this in a good way. I was driving down into Boise for the very first race of my adult life. Ever since we had moved to Boise from

Pullman, Washington, back in the '80s, this race had captured my attention. It was known as "the toughest race" back before it was in vogue to create grueling, impossible-sounding races. It was called "the Race to Robie Creek," and it's still a highly popular race in our area.

I had never dreamed I would be running this race myself, over a decade later. As soon as I realized I could run, even though I was in my late thirties, I started dreaming of running this race. I had enjoyed running hills back in Pullman, and as I mentioned earlier, dirt roads were a little piece of heaven to me. Living where we did, I had all I could ever hope for of both. Almost directly out our front door, heading out for a run, I had two choices: up or down. And if I chose down, it goes without saying that the way home would be up. There was no shin-shredding pavement to be found anywhere. Like I said, for me it was heaven on earth.

The first year I started running, I immediately wanted to do the Race to Robie Creek. My husband gave me a flat no. He had not been running, so he would not be in shape for the race. There would be men at the finish line, at the post-race party, and he didn't want me there without him. Of course, I knew this was not a concern, but he was the family decision-maker, and he let me know it wasn't happening. He told me I would be allowed to do it the following year because he would start running, too, and we would then be able to run it together, without the perils of me being left "unsupervised." (Oops, there I go. I told you I had given up being sarcastic, but I let that one slip out.)

As I progressed in my training, I realized that training for an extra year before attempting this race was a smart move. I learned what it was like to build a base of running, progressing slowly and steadily instead of going all out and injuring myself, as I had in high school and college. I still had my share of injuries because I had a lot to learn about running, but through the process, I learned how to manage and heal from them one by one, and how to avoid them in the future.

I didn't make the connection at the time, but looking back, I can see where my husband's resistance to my running came from. He thought it was his duty to run this race with me, and here I was going out running without him. I was getting ahead of him. I was doing it for the sheer love of running, the freedom and joy I felt when I was out there, and the exhilaration of watching myself steadily improve. To his way of thinking, it was disrespectful for me to go out running without him. I should wait until he found the time in his schedule, he felt like it, and the weather was conducive to running, and then we would go out together. Then he would be naturally stronger and faster than me, as was proper, and he could accompany me on my race.

But he didn't forbid me to run, so I ran. When he told me that running was my god, I knew that wasn't true. Running was bringing me closer to God and helping me to reawaken spiritually after a long drought. He also told me, "Running is your one joy in life." That wasn't true, either, but running was the one thing, more than anything else, that reawakened joy for me. It was unlocking the door to the prison I had trapped myself in. Running was setting me free.

Back to driving to that first Race to Robie Creek. My husband had long since given up on the idea that he was going to run it with me, but he was still running it and would be along shortly after I finished to accompany me to the post-race party.

I had dreamed of this race, perhaps on every run I had taken, for over a year. I was strong and fit, probably fitter than I had ever been my entire life. Except for a nagging knee injury, I felt fabulous. I was just about to turn thirty-nine.

But there in the car, fear started rushing in. What if I had bitten off more than I could chew? What if I couldn't finish? What if I were way slower than I thought I would be? I had friends who were excited for me. Would I be letting them down if I didn't do well?

Sitting there in the car, I realized the answer was no. My friends weren't happy for me because they thought I would get a good finish time. They were happy for me because I was happy. With that realization, all the pressure I felt suddenly melted away. *Nobody cares*. It doesn't mean anything, to anybody, whether I do well (by my own internal standard) in this race or not. Those who cared just wanted me to be happy.

Nobody who cared about me was going to laugh at me or ridicule me. Nobody was going to point a finger and say, "See, we knew you were a failure. We knew you wouldn't measure up."

I realized in that moment that this was a story I had carried with me since high school, when the guys on the track team couldn't believe how slow I was. They couldn't believe how anybody could possibly be that slow and still call it running. They weren't going to be there at the finish line at Robie Creek. In fact, twenty years later, my guess is they all burned themselves out in high school and college, and were now sitting on the couch, beer firmly in hand. Just a guess. But in any event, nobody was going to be there at the finish line to point fingers and laugh at me.

Nobody cares.

This idea was so freeing. At this race, I would be just another runner in a sea of runners with their own aspirations, fears, and doubts. Each one would run their own race and cross their own finish line. I couldn't run somebody else's race, and I didn't want to. We each have our own race to run, and that is true in all aspects of life.

I had plenty of naysayers in my life, including friends, neighbors, and family members. But I had gotten past caring about what they thought or said. I knew I was doing the very best thing for me. Ironically, the few people who were cheering me on were the people I thought I would be letting down if I didn't do well in my race. I didn't know I felt that way until sitting in the car that day. But no, I wouldn't be letting anyone down if I didn't make it to the finish line. I might hear "I told you so" from the naysayers, but no one who cared would be disappointed in me.

FREEDOM FROM APPROVAL SEEKING

What was so freeing about this realization was that, suddenly, I knew this was only for me. In my growing-up years, I had needed the approval of others to validate myself. It went beyond wanting to be one of the cool kids. I had already given up hope of that. And that's only a surface need. It was the need to know I was okay as a human being, in other people's eyes; that was my true felt need. I think we all have a need for approval from others, whether parents, other family members, or friends. When we don't feel we have that approval, it can lead us down the path to those addictive behaviors we've been talking about.

Let's take a look at that for a moment. This is one of those "in-the-jar" things. When we've been so caught up in approval seeking for most of our lives, it's hard to separate ourselves from that line of thinking. It's second nature, like breathing. It's been part of my growing-up process in the past few years to put all of that behind me. I can see I still have farther to go in that process, but at least I can recognize it, examine it, and lay it to rest when it rears its ugly head.

The ramifications of this understanding are huge. Can you imagine what it would be like to be living your own life, without worrying about being judged by others? Everything we're so worried that they are thinking about us is a story we've made up in our own heads. When those people express their disapproval directly to us, that's their story, not ours. We are free to evaluate and take their words into consideration. If they fit, and they suit us, we can wear them. Or we can set them aside. But we don't have to own them, if they don't belong to us.

Pay attention to your thoughts and you may start to see how many of them are taken up with stories about what others are thinking about us. The truth is they're so busy concocting their own stories about what others are thinking about them that they don't have time to think all those thoughts about you. They are in their own world, just as you are in yours. Isn't that a freeing thought? Wouldn't it be amazing just to be present, living your own life, moment by moment, instead of trying to live others' lives and think their thoughts for them?

Even though my clients and I dive deep into their stories, my job as a coach is not to be a problem solver or advice giver. When my clients come to me seeking advice or answers to their dilemmas, I always try to point them back to what they already know—to the answers that are already inside of them. The foundation we lay of a new way of thinking about life gives them a whole new way of approaching problems. I call my program "Celebrate the New You" because that's exactly what we learn to do. When we learn to break free from the old ways of thinking that have been keeping us stuck for all these years, there is a lot to celebrate. The old ways of thinking are still there because, after all, we've been living with them for a lifetime. But as my clients progress through the program and their understanding of a new way starts to emerge, I help them apply it to what they're struggling with in the here and now. With practice, this muscle gets strengthened, and the new way becomes automatic.

Those who see my program, Celebrate the New You, as being centered around weight loss will be confused. What does all this have to do with losing weight? New members in my program quickly see it is not really about losing weight. Weight loss is a byproduct of being free. Freedom starts in our minds. When we are engaged in seeking the approval of others, we are not free. Our mission together is to set you free from every roadblock and obstacle that comes up in your thinking so you will experience a clarity of mind you've never had before.

What if the only obstacles you faced only existed in your own mind? What if there was absolutely nothing standing in your way to reaching a life of freedom? What if your success was inevitable?

QUESTIONS FOR REFLECTION

What are some ways you can start applying the idea that "nothing happens to me; it only happens for me" in your life?

_____
_____
_____
_____

How can you remind yourself to start looking for the lesson in every circumstance?

_____
_____
_____
_____

Are you ready to start making the choice to be the victor? What will that look like for you?

_____
_____
_____
_____

Chapter 8

Taking It with You

I don't know how many books I've read that promised they would change my life. Did they? I think some of them did, if I define changing my life as the myriad small breakthroughs and transformations I've experienced along the way. Certainly many important realizations have come to me through reading books. Others have come to me through my life experiences and how I chose to look at them. And still others have come from direct coaching and mentorship that I have received. All the experiences, all the learnings, and all the breakthroughs, big and small, have added up to the place I'm in now.

And there is so, so much more to come. I haven't arrived, and I don't plan on ever arriving in this lifetime. But every year, I grow to love this journey of life I'm on a little bit more. Maybe even a lot more. This is an amazing life we are living. It's amazing that you are here, alive, right now, experiencing this beautiful life.

A while back, my sister Terri did some digging into our family tree. It was a meaningful time for us because our aunt had just passed away, and her passing represented the end of an era for our family. I won't go into all the details, but it was a time of reflection for my sister and me. As we looked over one branch of our family history, I was impressed to see how many of our ancestors had come over to this country across the Atlantic in rickety boats in the seventeenth and eighteenth centuries. So many of them had only one child, or only one who survived into adulthood. My great-grandfather died of the 1918 flu when my grandmother was just three years old.

The odds of me—or you—being here to live this incredible, beautiful life are astronomical. That is true for every single one of us on this planet. Being here is a miracle. Let that sink in for a moment. Are you ready to start living this amazing life you have been given? Are you ready to let go of the shame that has kept you hidden away as a fraction of who you were really meant to be? What if there was so much more inside you just waiting to be expressed? All the guilt, the anger, the bitterness, and everything else that has held you back—are you ready to let it all go? Because it's a choice. If I were to guess, I would say the underlying emotion behind all these other emotions and beliefs you're hanging onto is fear. It takes courage to step into your true self. Most women I talk to would rather stay in the fear. It is all they have ever known, and ironically enough, it is the place that feels safe. They don't realize it's fear that's keeping them stuck, but in many cases, that's what it boils down to. They would rather hide behind all the reasons why now is not the time and tomorrow would be so much better to start living the life they want for themselves.

But not you. I encourage you to do what it takes to start winning in life. Leave behind the regret, the fear, the shame, and the guilt, and start learning what it means to be free. You are worth it. Don't worry about how long or difficult the road is ahead of you. Take the first step. Then you will see your way to taking the next step. The farther you have to go, the more courage it takes. But the farther you have to travel, the more you will inspire yourself when you see you're making progress toward your goals.

Imagine yourself being that success story that others aspire to. How good will that feel? That victory is yours for the taking. But you have to learn how not to give up on yourself. You can do that one simple act of taking the next step, whatever that is for you, and then the next. If you don't allow yourself to give up, you will get there. You will achieve your goals. It doesn't come by beating yourself up. It doesn't come by shaming yourself into shape. It comes through learning to value and love yourself, along with caring for yourself in a way you have never done before. It comes through picking yourself back up and carrying on toward your dream.

And that's a rare thing in our world. You will be inspiring others long before you have reached your goals. The small, consistent steps you are taking will start to be noticed. Don't let that scare you. Don't let it cause you to self-sabotage or retreat. Just accept it for what it is. Whether you are comfortable in this place or not, you are stepping into the position of role model for others. I don't say that to put any pressure on you. You are doing this for you, not for others. Your own missteps are yours alone. You don't have to feel like you're in the spotlight. This is your journey, not anyone else's. All I'm saying is others will start to notice you are coming at this with a whole new attitude and perspective. And that new way of being is contagious.

I've had more than a few women tell me they do just fine on their weight-loss journey until someone notices they've lost weight and makes a congratulatory comment to them. On hearing that comment, they will immediately revert back into their old ways and gain all the weight right back. Many of us fear failure, but even more debilitating, we can fear success. Something inside us wants to hold us back and keep us playing small. To reach for success is stepping into the unknown. It can feel like a great abyss. Our fear keeps us from stepping into the new identity of someone in charge of her life. Yet, although the fear of success is real, it can be a difficult fear to comprehend. Who doesn't want to be successful? Yet many of us shrink back from being noticed in any way. We would rather just blend into the background. It feels safer that way.

IT'S TIME

I'm here to tell you it's time. It's time to break through all the fear and every barrier that's standing in your way and rise up into your own greatness. Yes, it's scary. But the first step into freedom can often be the scariest. Once we've picked up a little momentum, it starts to take less and less effort to continue moving ourselves forward. By the way, here's one of the biggest and most life-changing lessons my clients learn: the idea that this journey is "hard" is actually just a story we've become accustomed to telling ourselves through years of trying and failing. We learn in my program how to turn that story around and make it easy on ourselves to win. Part of that new identity we take on is learning how to accept our success as a natural outflow of stepping into our greatness.

Now the world gets to experience you. You get to experience being unashamedly you. You get to experience what it's like to be free.

And you will never want to put yourself back in prison once you've truly experienced what it is to be free.

Some of the women reading this book will take what I've given them here and run with it. But just as I never could have escaped the trap of emotional addiction I was in by reading a book or googling for answers, you may be feeling like you need a tour guide on your journey. You need a mentor.

The friends I turned to for help when I was trapped in the prison of addiction were kind, compassionate, and helpful. But they were often at a loss to know how best to help me. I couldn't have broken free without their encouragement and support. But, ultimately, I had to figure it out for myself. I know I would have found the answers much more quickly had I been able to find the expert guidance I needed.

Now, I understand that the women I coach every day do not have the tools, the system, or the support they need to break free. They could be surrounded by caring people, but those people aren't equipped to help in the way these women desperately need. They could scour the internet all day long, every day, and not find the answers that an expert who understands addiction can pinpoint for them in just moments. This is not about gathering more information. If it were, all our problems would be solved, because in the history of the world we've never before had access to the vast quantities of information at our fingertips right now. What is keeping you stuck is on the inside. You won't find it in the latest diet plan. You can't read the label when you're inside the jar. You need someone who cares, who can read the label, and who can give you the guidance you need to get out of that stuck place.

As much as I want this book to transform your life, I know a book can never accomplish that. It's possible that applying the information in this book (or in any one of dozens of books) deeply and reflectively to your current thinking may be transformational. But the truth is, we almost always need an outsider's perspective into our thought processes to understand what's going on inside our own heads. I'm not a mind reader, but understanding what's behind the stories that my clients share with me can help me to help them turn their thinking around very quickly.

We can read all the right words, but until we take that extra step of seeing how it applies right here and right now to our own thought processes, we're going to stay stuck. It's my job, for my clients anyway, to help them get unstuck. If I give them advice, or try to solve their problems for them, they're going to stay stuck. The last thing I want is to make them dependent on me. I'm a coach, and it's my job as a coach to bring out the best in you.

I always tell my clients I'm like the training wheels to their bicycle. If they stick with it long enough and are willing to pick themselves back up after the inevitable crashes, they will learn to ride. Yeah, you might be a little beat up. You might wake up stiff and sore the next morning. But the freedom of riding that bicycle, the feeling of the wind in your face, is worth it all once you've made the shift into that freedom. My goal for my clients is independence, where they know they don't need me anymore. And that's what a good coach will do for you.

You can join all the weight-loss and dieting programs this world has to offer, but those are only addressing the symptoms to the problem. If you really want to be free, you need a different path. Freedom starts in your thinking. I can hear instantly, whenever I'm talking to a client on the phone, the places where she is stuck in her thinking. Simply pointing it out to her won't do any good. That will just be more advice giving, and it will only serve to keep her in that stuck place and make her feel a little bit worse about herself that she is still there.

Once again, we're each stuck inside our own jar, unable to read the label that's plain to see from the outside of the jar. I believe we all need a coach to help us read the label. A coach brings that outsider perspective, comes alongside us and takes us by the hand, and helps us reach that next level.

Today, I just can't get enough of personal development and growth. For me, these days, this almost always involves a coach. My quest to be the very best version of me is not because I want to be better than anyone else. In fact, I would love to take the whole world with me on my journey. The key I have learned is to turn every "I can't" into "How can I?" and just get curious. How can I make this work? It's an empowering question.

I used the example of training wheels a few moments ago. In reality, it's not the training wheels that teach us to ride a bike. Training wheels teach us how to rely on the training wheels. I had the training wheels on for quite a while and never learned how to ride. Only when my dad took the training wheels off and ran alongside me, holding onto the seat, did I finally learn. Pretty soon, he was running alongside with his hand off the seat, without me even realizing it. I got a little ways ahead and saw he wasn't there. Crash! Ah, but there was a new understanding in that crash. I had done it. I had balanced on those two thin wheels all by myself while propelling myself forward. Pretty soon, my dad was helping me get started, and I was leaving him behind. I was riding! Now to learn to steer, and to brake, while keeping myself upright. I'm sure I had more than a few scrapes to show from that first day of riding, but I had done it. I was free.

I'm telling you that you need a coach. "But Lynn," you may argue, "look at how far you got without a coach. You learned how to set yourself free. Why can't I do the same?"

I've got a few reasons for you. First, all of these small realizations in my life happened over many years. The understandings were slow and gradual. They seem fast because I've condensed the years of learnings into a book you're sitting here reading now. You have the bird's eye view of my life. A coach can take what you need to learn and reveal it to you in a way that will make sense to you, and knock years, if not decades, off your growth process. If you want to make real progress and start living your life instead of being locked away in a prison, gradually chipping away at the lock with a butter knife, I recommend you invest in a coach.

A coach can unlock that door for you in a matter of minutes and help set you free. This isn't a perfect analogy (no analogy really is) because there are likely many things holding you back, and we only work with one thing at a time. But as you learn to recognize the thought processes that are the locks on your prison door, they start to unlock for you much more quickly. You learn the combination that you can keep applying to different situations to get you out of those stuck places. You make friends with the new ways of thinking, and they start to become the default. When you learn to live at peace in your own mind and you're filled with gratitude as the default, then all the negativity, worry, and fear become more and more incongruent. It starts to not feel right to live there anymore. You have a new address.

Second, I did have help for the one deepest prison I was locked in. A lot of help. I leaned hard on my friends. One of those friends was a pastor's wife, so she may have spoken with more authority than my other friends, but mercifully for me, they all had personal experience dealing with the very problem I was facing. They had all navigated those same waters successfully. All three of them held me in wisdom, compassion, and love, along with boatloads of patience.

And third, I have learned to be resourceful. I used to believe that investing in a coach was completely out of reach for me. Now I know that's not true. Now I surround myself with strategically chosen mentors and coaches to get me where I want to go in every area of my life in which I want to make real progress. As of today, I have a swim coach, a book-writing coach (hence the book you are holding in your hands or reading on your computer, because without Christine it would probably still be floating around in my mind as a good idea), a coach to train me in how to be a better coach, a coach with a PhD in organizational psychology, and all the business and mindset mentoring, coaching, and guidance I could ever want through a program I am a member of. Maybe I go a little crazy on coaches because I was told I would never succeed. I'm not sure. But one thing I do know: I've learned how to dream big and throw all my energy into reaching for my dreams. Guess what? I'm worth it. My confidence is growing, little by little. It doesn't happen all in one day, but it doesn't even matter how quickly or slowly I get to my finish line. I'm in love with the journey. I'm in love with the growth. I'm in love with being free.

MAKE YOUR SUCCESS INEVITABLE

Really, it all boils down to mindset. My mindset and my belief that my success is inevitable are growing stronger by the day. That is not by accident. That is by intention. The reason I have something to give you is I am continuously investing in myself.

When I encourage women to invest in themselves, I know I am investing far, far more in myself than I am asking of them. I see the greatness in them that they can't see. There is so much potential locked away in each one of us. I know if I hadn't taken each step to invest in myself at the next level, I would still be in my own little prison to this day. Probably not that same one I was locked away in twenty-five years ago. I would have found a new one. I would have found a new way of medicating myself to cope with all the pain I was in. I would have kept myself playing small.

Now, I feel as though I've climbed up a hill, and I'm standing at the ridgeline and taking in all the vistas in front of me. There is so much more to life than we can see from down in the valley. And I want more. I'm calling back to you in your valley to let you know the view's amazing up here. I'm not here to manipulate or convince you into joining me on the journey. But I want more for you, because I see what's possible. I see that the sky's the limit—it is for me, and I know it is for you, too. I don't care if you're 150 or 200 pounds overweight and you've given up all but the tiniest flicker of hope. I don't care if the TV has been your best friend for the past ten years. I don't care if you can barely make it from the couch to the kitchen without feeling like you're dragging yourself there. I don't care if you've tried every diet plan under the sun.

There is hope for you. There is the possibility of freedom. You can start to dream again, and you can begin to live into those dreams with intention. You can take the next step.

Reading a book isn't going to get you there. It never does. If I gave you that impression, I apologize. *Taking action* on the book's message, however, can absolutely set you free. My hope in writing this book is to awaken that little spark of hope in you, to get you dreaming again, and to get you started down the path toward that beautiful life of freedom that awaits you.

QUESTIONS FOR REFLECTION

What does it mean to you to be resourceful?
_____
_____
_____
_____

What fears are holding you back?
_____
_____
_____
_____

What is the next step for you?
_____
_____
_____
_____

Are you ready to be free?
_____
_____
_____
_____

A Final Note:

Opportunity over Impossibility

I just gave you a list of some of the ways I am currently investing in myself. Maybe you're thinking, *Must be nice, Lynn, to have all that money to invest in yourself like that. As for me, I'm broke.*

I spent much of my adult life living well below the poverty line. I never considered us poor, but I did learn to be very resourceful. I wasn't calling it this back then, but I continually had to learn to pick myself up out of my scarcity mindset and put on an opportunity mindset. When I saw something that was going to move me forward into a better life for myself and my family, I found a way to make it happen, even if it seemed impossible. Faith over fear. Opportunity over impossibility. Small shifts in thinking make a world of difference.

We all can hold the belief that we're in some special circumstance that prevents us from climbing out of our own special pit we're stuck in. It's my belief there is a way out, no matter how deep your hole is. Every time I invest in myself, I feel that fear rising up. What if I'm making a mistake? What if it doesn't pay off, and I end up homeless and destitute? It has been a stretch every single time I've made a significant decision to invest in myself.

I'm not talking about "shelf help." There are all kinds of purchases we make that we don't think twice about. Some of them may move us forward a little bit, and some never even make it out of the cellophane they came wrapped in. The reason they don't make much of a dent is precisely because those investments *didn't* scare us. They didn't move the needle on our subconscious mind's reading of danger ahead. We made the purchase, didn't even feel it, felt good we had done something toward our progress (whether it did anything for us or not), and then moved on. We all have done it, if we look honestly at it.

Just as I told you I didn't really work at the classes I thought would be easy and got the best grades in the ones I went into scared, it's the same thing here. Making a significant decision to break out of your prison should be scary. We don't like to be scared. We like to be comfortable. But that's precisely why you are where you are right now. You've kept yourself comfortable, and in the case of your health, comfort is deadly.

But what is your life worth to you? Can you really put a price tag on it? I'm not asking you these questions for my own benefit. What I'm suggesting is that you decide, right now, that you are going to pay the price to win, no matter the cost. You are a woman of tremendous worth. That has nothing to do with money, but the money is a symbol of what you are worth to you. I only work with women who understand they are worth investing in. I only work with women who are 100 percent committed to a brand spankin' new life for themselves. They are sick and tired of the old, worn-out paths, and they're ready for a new way. More importantly, they understand they haven't been living their life. They're tired of being in prison. They are ready to be free.

We all have our own obstacles—mental, logistical, physical, circumstantial, or otherwise—to overcome. Our ability to climb over, dig under, or maneuver our way around somehow, and find a way to move ourselves forward into our freedom determines whether or not we will obtain that freedom. I look at how far I've come out of poverty and hopelessness and despair. I look back through eyes of wonder. If I had tried to climb the mountain all in one leap, I would have crashed on the rocks. I did it the way we climb every mountain in front of us: one small step at a time. As I write this, I am filled with nothing but gratitude. I hope you will find a way to make that next small step. Not because it will change my life, but because it will absolutely change every single day of the rest of yours.

The value of your life is incomprehensible. It's a miracle that you're even here. And you're here at just the right time. You only get one chance on this incredible planet, and that one shot is too precious to spend being stuck. You were meant for more. Don't let anything hold you back from reaching for the freedom to be all you were meant to be.

My sincerest wish is for you to start living your life. I hope you will give yourself permission to start being you. Not the you hidden beneath layers of stories, or shame or guilt or fear, but the real you. I hope the world—your world—will get to experience the beauty and the miracle of you. The you who is free of addiction and fear and regret, and is living in joy, abundance, and gratitude. The world will be happy to meet the real, amazing you. You have a place here. There is no need to hide anymore.

Acknowledgments

I am grateful to so many. My sister Terri gave me my powerful "why" to build Be Fit Beyond Fifty. She's also been my most helpful sounding board for all aspects of my business. My son Sean has been a huge encouragement and has provided me with a lot of the "how." All my adult kids have been an inspiration. I am immensely grateful to them for being awesome humans and bringing so much joy into my life. My husband Ross has believed in me and been my most avid supporter. Debi, our caregiver extraordinaire, has taken a tremendous load off my shoulders to enable me to do what I do. I couldn't have gotten by without a whole lot of help from my friends and family. Thank you to each one of you.

I have been influenced by the work of so many, but the two who stand out in the forefront of my mind are Byron Katie and Dr. Benjamin Hardy. I have allowed Byron Katie's work to sink down into the core of my being. Without her, this book certainly wouldn't exist. I am grateful for the opportunity to be a member of Ben Hardy's Amp Platinum coaching program, but his influence on my thinking has preceded that membership by several years. My weekly check-ins with Natasha as a member of Amp have been tremendously helpful.

Nick and Megan Unsworth of Life on Fire played an important part in helping me be set free from my limiting beliefs and stories that were holding me back. Through Life on Fire, I became acquainted with Christine Gail, who ultimately became my book coach. She knew how to lovingly push me forward in all the right ways to bring this book to fruition. She brought me into contact with my amazing editor, Tyler Tichelaar of Superior Book Productions, who has been a pleasure to work with and who has helped me see the blind spots in my writing.

I can't begin to describe what being a part of Clients on Demand has done for me. Russ Ruffino, Marc von Musser, Jessie Torres, and all the rest of the COD team and fellow members are day by day helping me turn all my dreams into reality. I am continually astounded by the work they do and how they pour themselves into others.

And finally, I am beyond grateful to the One who told me, "I will never leave you nor forsake you."

About the Author

LYNN WEIMAR, MSN, has turned her passion for fitness, particularly running, into a mission to transform the lives of women beyond fifty who struggle with emotional eating, food addictions, and obesity. Having struggled with self-image and addiction issues herself, she has combined her previous healing process and mindset work with her experience as an RN and research as an MSN to bring hope and freedom to both her audience and her private clients.

Lynn is the founder of Be Fit Beyond Fifty, and *Be Free Beyond Fifty* is her first book. Besides running, she loves swimming, biking, dabbling in languages, and learning chess. She is very proud and grateful to be rocking her sixties and is dreaming of spending her golden years traveling the world and competing in Ironman triathlons. She lives in Cascade, Idaho, with her husband, Ross, Ross's dad, Bob, her adult son, Sean, and their rescue parakeets, Puff and Rainbow.

Be Set Free to Live Your Best Life

Are you locked in a prison of food addictions, emotional eating, obesity, shame, or regret?

Are you ready to be free?

Lynn Weimar's exclusive coaching program, Celebrate the New You, picks up where *Be Free Beyond Fifty* leaves off, taking you on a journey to freedom through inner transformation.

Lynn believes that to reach our optimal lives, we need a mentor to help guide us there. Lynn's program is designed to carefully remove every obstacle that is holding *you* back so you can say goodbye to dieting forever and heal your relationship with food once and for all. More than that, you will learn how to truly value and love yourself, create a powerful vision of your new life of freedom, and live into that vision day by day.

One of the best ways to connect with Lynn is through joining her free masterclass, Five Simple Shifts to Eliminate Emotional Eating. You can do so through this URL: masterclass.befitbeyondfifty.com

Are you ready to be free? Your dream is worth it.

To learn more, go to BeFitBeyondFifty.com
or email lynn@befitbeyondfifty.com